The Physician's Guide to Eye Care

How to Diagnose
How to Treat
When to Refer

American Academy of Ophthalmology
655 Beach Street
P.O. Box 7424
San Francisco, CA 94120-7424

Academy Staff

Kathryn A. Hecht, EdD, Vice President, Clinical Education
Hal Straus, Publications Manager
Margaret Petela, Managing Editor
Pearl C. Vapnek, Medical Editor

Cover illustration: "The Eye Puzzle," by Lewis Calver.
Copyright © 1983 Retina Foundation of the Southwest,
Dallas, Texas. Reprinted with permission of the Retina Foundation
of the Southwest, Dallas, Texas.

Interior illustrations: Biomedical Communications,
University of Michigan, Ann Arbor

The Physician's Guide to Eye Care

Jonathan D. Trobe, MD

Professor of Ophthalmology
Associate Professor of Neurology
University of Michigan

Developed in cooperation with

American Academy of Family Physicians
American Academy of Pediatrics
American College of Emergency Physicians
American College of Physicians

American Academy of Ophthalmology

Library of Congress Cataloging-in-Publication Data

Trobe, Jonathan D., 1943-
    The physician's guide to eye care / Jonathan D. Trobe.
        p.   cm.
    Includes bibliographical references and index.
    ISBN 1-56055-073-2
    1. Ophthalmology. 2. Primary care (Medicine) I. Title.
    [DNLM: 1. Eye Diseases.   WW 140 T843p 1993]
RE48.T76   1993
617.7—dc20
DNLM/DLC
for Library of Congress   93-9068
                                                                CIP

97 96 95 94   5 4 3 2 1

Contents

Chapter 4   The Red Eye   41

Chapter 5   Ophthalmic Trauma   65

Chapter 6   Systemic Diseases   **77**

Chapter 7   Ophthalmic Medications   101

Chapter 8   Systemic Medications   119

Chapter 9   Principal Conditions   129

Appendix A   Common Questions From Patients   161

Appendix B   Illustrated Ophthalmic Anatomy   167

Appendix C   Annotated Resources   173

Index   177

Close-Ups

Preface

Whether you are a pediatrician, internist, or family, emergency, or other primary care physician, eye care problems constitute a significant part of your medical practice. In searching for books to help you manage these problems, you have probably encountered very few volumes, and those were most likely written from an ophthalmologist's point of view.

This book is different. Both the topics and the text format are the result of surveys of, discussions with, and extensive reviews by physicians from several primary care specialties. These physicians recommended that a manual on eye care delineate the distinctive and the collaborative roles of primary care physicians and ophthalmologists in eye care. They also suggested that the book provide easy access to practical information in concise language and through plentiful illustration.

Based on these recommendations, this text does not follow the standard disease-by-structure organization. Rather, it is organized around the most common clinical challenges:

□ How to perform an ophthalmic screening examination (Chapter 1)

□ How often to screen the asymptomatic patient (Chapter 2)

□ How to interpret common ophthalmic symptoms and signs (Chapter 3)

□ How to manage the red eye (Chapter 4)

□ How to handle eye trauma (Chapter 5)

□ How to evaluate ophthalmic signs and symptoms that accompany specific systemic illnesses, and when to consult an ophthalmologist (Chapter 6)

□ How to decide whether symptoms are due to the effects of ocular medications (Chapter 7)

□ How to determine whether systemic medications might harm the eyes (Chapter 8)

Chapter 9, "Principal Conditions," offers short, informative articles on the 15 ophthalmic entities identified in surveys as being those most frequently encountered. For instant reference, each article is preceded by "At a Glance," a list of facts from the article that are most important for the primary care physician to know.

Appendix A helps you answer the questions patients ask most frequently, about everything from eyeglasses and contact lenses to the effects of "overusing" the eyes. A visual overview of ophthalmic anatomy is presented in six full-color illustrations in Appendix B. For further information, Appendix C lists annotated resources, from introductory texts to specialized references, including videotape and slide programs.

This book offers several special features intended to enhance its value as a ready reference on your office bookshelf:

- Step-by-step process descriptions, illustrated in color, that simplify screening and treatment methods
- Lists and tables that highlight important clinical findings
- Suggested specific questions that you might ask patients as part of the ocular and medical history-taking
- "Close-Up" vignettes that present important related clinical topics
- Color photographs of major entities
- Complete index for quick and easy cross-referencing

Because this volume is organized for practical use rather than as a student textbook, related aspects of a given entity or clinical topic may be covered in numerous places throughout the book. Readers are encouraged to take full advantage of the thorough index.

This publication is the result of a cooperative effort to bridge the information gap between ophthalmologists and other generalist and specialist physicians who share the responsibility for patients' eye health. If it helps you to manage clinical problems with greater confidence and success, it will have fulfilled its purpose.

Acknowledgments

The author wishes to acknowledge and thank the following individuals who contributed to the development and production of this book.

For assistance in developing the manuscript:

American Academy of Ophthalmology, Professional Liaison Committee
Richard L. Abbott, MD; Keith D. Carter, MD; Elizabeth J. Cohen, MD;
Susan H. Day, MD; Andrew S. Farber, MD; Marilyn C. Kincaid, MD;
Jane D. Kivlin, MD; Gary Arsham, MD (Consultant)

For review and valuable critique of the manuscript:

American Academy of Ophthalmology
George W. Blankenship, MD; Thomas A. Deutsch, MD; Dan B. Jones, MD;
Scott M. MacRae, MD; Richard P. Mills, MD; Louis D. Pizzarello, MD

American Academy of Family Physicians
Eugene Felmar, MD; David Hoff, MD

American Academy of Pediatrics, Ophthalmology Section
Edward G. Buckley, MD; Earl R. Crouch, MD; Gary R. Diamond, MD;
Frederick J. Elsas, MD; Mark J. Greenwald, MD; Stanley I. Hand, MD;
David A. Hiles, MD; Jane D. Kivlin, MD; Graham E. Quinn, MD;
Michael T. Trese, MD; Kenneth W. Wright, MD

*American Academy of Pediatrics, Committee on Practice
and Ambulatory Care Medicine*
Roger F. Suchyta, MD

American College of Emergency Physicians
Roland B. Clark, MD

American College of Physicians
F. Daniel Duffy, MD

The author also wishes to thank Ellyn Glazer Cohen, PhD, Margaret Petela, and
Pearl C. Vapnek for editorial assistance; Christopher J. Burke for developing and
producing illustrations; and Csaba L. Martonyi for help in selecting photographs.

The Physician's Guide to Eye Care

How to Diagnose
How to Treat
When to Refer

CHAPTER I

The Screening Examination

The ophthalmic screening examination is used in two circumstances: for periodic evaluation of patients who do not have ophthalmic symptoms (Chapter 2), and for evaluation of patients who do have ophthalmic symptoms (Chapters 3 to 5).

Components of the Examination

The ophthalmic screening examination has six basic components:

☐ Visual acuity

☐ Confrontation visual fields

☐ External examination

☐ Pupillary examination

☐ Motility and alignment examination

☐ Ophthalmoscopic examination

The Close-Up "Equipment for the Ophthalmic Screening Examination" groups the basic equipment by component of the examination.

Visual Acuity

Measuring visual acuity is usually the first step in the ophthalmic screening examination. Although the Snellen test is the most familiar, various other methods have been devised to measure or estimate visual acuity in young children,

CLOSE-UP

EQUIPMENT FOR THE OPHTHALMIC SCREENING EXAMINATION

Procedure	Equipment
Visual acuity	Snellen eye chart, near vision card (adults); picture chart or tumbling E chart (preliterate children)
Confrontation visual fields	None
External examination	Penlight, fluorescein strips, topical anesthetic, cobalt-blue light
Pupillary examination	Penlight, pupil gauge (may be found on the near vision card)
Motility and alignment examination	Penlight, distance fixation target
Ophthalmoscopic examination	Direct ophthalmoscope, 2.5% phenylephrine (for dilating pupils)

mentally deficient patients, and individuals with extremely low vision. The Close-Up "Boundaries of Normal Visual Acuity" lists acceptable visual acuity test results for normal individuals in three age groups.

Distance Vision (Snellen) Test

The Snellen chart displays lines of block letters of diminishing size, each defined according to the distance at which the line of letters can be read by a person with normal acuity (Figure 1-1). For example, the 20/100 line is the smallest line of print that a person with normal visual acuity could read correctly at a testing distance of 100 feet.

Snellen visual acuity is expressed by a numerator and a denominator, but the notation is not a fraction. The numerator is the testing distance (20 feet); the denominator is the smallest line of print the patient can read at that testing distance.

To perform the Snellen test, do the following:

1. Position the patient at the designated distance (ideally, 20 feet) from a well-illuminated Snellen chart.

2. With the patient wearing the customary eyeglasses or contact lenses used for distance viewing, test each eye separately, being careful to completely occlude (but not compress) the eye not being tested.

3. For each eye, record the smallest line of print the patient can read. If most letters on a line are correctly identified, give the patient credit for that line.

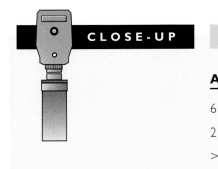

CLOSE-UP

BOUNDARIES OF NORMAL VISUAL ACUITY	
Age Group	**Normal Visual Acuity**
6 months to 3 years	Ability to fix and follow face, toy, or light
2 to 5 years	20/40 or better; 2-line difference between eyes
>5 years	20/30 or better; 2-line difference between eyes

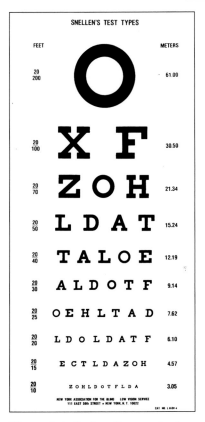

Figure 1-1 Snellen distance visual acuity chart. In the fractions at the left of each line of letters, the numerator specifies the testing distance and the denominator specifies the letter size in relation to letters on the 20/20 line. Thus, the 20/100 letters are 5 times larger than the 20/20 letters. (Courtesy W.K. Kellogg Eye Center, University of Michigan.)

4. If acuity is poorer than the largest letter (either 20/200 or 20/400), have the patient approach the chart as close as necessary to read the largest letter correctly. If the viewing distance is 5 feet, the patient's acuity is recorded as 5/200 or 5/400, depending on the size of the largest letter.

Near Vision Test

The near vision test is used to assess reading vision and to measure visual acuity when distance vision cannot be tested (Figure 1-2). The method is identical to the Snellen test, except that the near vision card is held at the specified viewing distance (usually indicated on the near vision card as 14 inches from the eyes). As a test of visual acuity, this method is less accurate than the Snellen test for two reasons: (1) even a slight misestimation of testing distance will cause an incorrect measurement of acuity; and (2) the acuity measurement will be overestimated in uncorrected myopia and underestimated in uncorrected presbyopia. However, it is an acceptable and practical substitute when distance visual acuity cannot be measured.

Low-Vision Tests

If the patient cannot see the largest Snellen letter, measure acuity for each eye separately by one of the following methods, listed in order of decreasing visual function.

1. Counting-fingers acuity: Ask the patient to count the number of fingers you hold up at a specified distance, generally between 1 and 5 feet. Record the distance at which the patient successfully counts fingers (eg, CF 4 feet). If the patient is unsuccessful, perform hand-movements acuity testing.

2. Hand-movements acuity: Ask the patient to distinguish your horizontal from vertical hand motions at 1 foot. Record a positive response as HM. If the patient is unsuccessful, perform light-perception acuity testing.

3. Light-perception acuity: Ask whether the patient can see a bright light shined directly into the eyes. Record the result either as LP (light perception) or NLP (no light perception).

Figure 1-2 Near vision test. A less accurate but practical alternative to the Snellen distance visual acuity test. The card must be held as close to 14 inches from the eye as possible.

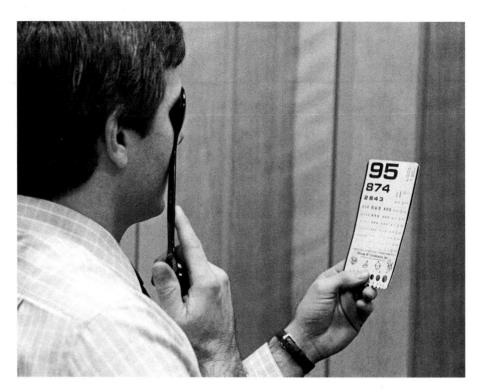

Fixation and Following

For children between 6 months and 2 years of age and for mentally deficient individuals, test visual function with the fixation-and-following method.

1. Observe the patient first with both of the patient's eyes open, then with one eye occluded at a time to determine whether the patient stares at (fixates) a stationary target (face, toy, or light) and pursues (follows) a moving target at arm's length.

2. If the patient is unable to perform this test, record the result as abnormal.

Picture Chart

Use the picture chart to test visual acuity in children between 2 and 4 years of age and in moderately mentally deficient individuals who cannot be tested with the tumbling E chart (see below) (Figure 1-3).

1. Ask the patient to identify standard pictures of diminishing size on a chart 20 feet away. A mute individual may be given an identical array of the pictures on cards and instructed to identify the distant picture by pointing to the identical one in the array. A scaled-down version is available for lap-distance testing (14 inches).

2. Record the measurement as for Snellen testing.

Tumbling E Chart

Use the tumbling E chart with children between 3 and 5 years of age and with mute, illiterate, or mildly mentally deficient individuals (Figure 1-4). This test is more accurate than the picture chart.

1. Ask the patient to identify, from 20 feet, the orientations of the letter E of diminishing size and various orientations by pointing the hand in the direction of the spokes of the E's. A scaled-down version is available for lap-distance testing (14 inches).

2. Record the measurement as for Snellen testing.

Common Causes of Visual Acuity Abnormalities

☐ Refractive disorder

☐ Amblyopia

☐ Corneal abrasion, corneal infection

☐ Cataract

☐ Age-related macular degeneration

☐ Optic neuritis, ischemic optic neuropathy

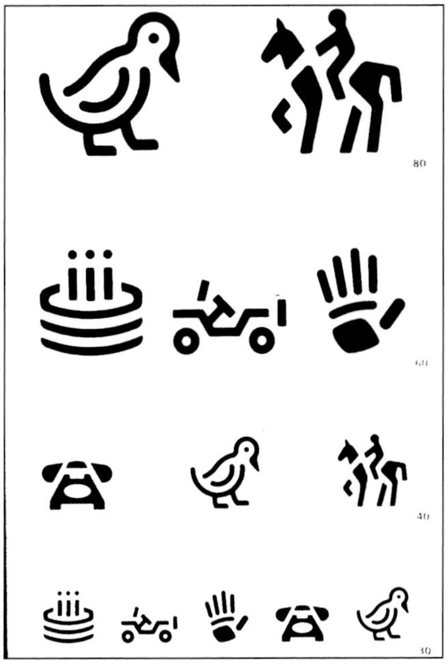

Figure 1-3 Picture chart. Used to test visual acuity in preliterate children aged 2 to 4 years and in moderately mentally deficient adults. Available for both distance and near testing.

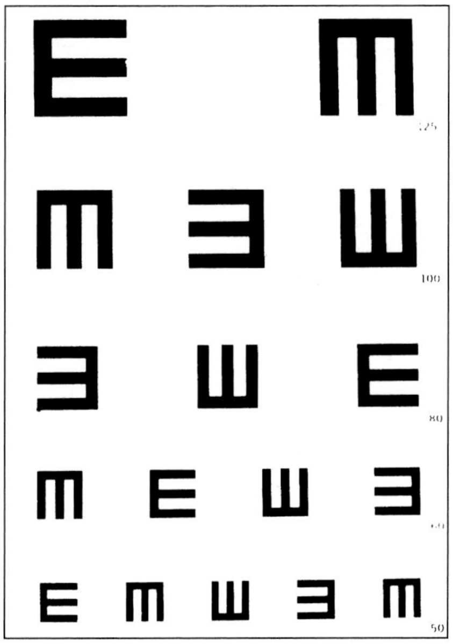

Figure 1-4 Tumbling E chart. A more quantitative alternative to picture cards for testing visual acuity in preliterate children aged 3 to 5 years and in mute, illiterate, or mildly mentally deficient adults. Available for both distance and near testing.

Confrontation Visual Fields

Confrontation visual field testing measures the patient's ability to identify large targets with peripheral vision. This test generally detects only gross visual pathway disturbances.

1. Sit directly in front of the patient, at a distance of 2 to 3 feet.

2. Close your right eye and have the patient cover his left eye.

3. Ask the patient to stare into your left eye. Check that your eye is positioned directly opposite the patient's eye.

4. Position your hand in a plane midway between the patient and yourself.

5. Sequentially display one or two fingers in each quadrant of the visual field (nasal superior and inferior, temporal superior and inferior) approximately 10 inches from fixation, and ask the patient to identify how many fingers you are displaying (Figure 1-5).

6. If the patient fails to identify fingers in one or more quadrants, record this as an abnormality. If the patient correctly identifies fingers in all quadrants, move to the next step, which is intended to help detect more subtle visual field deficits.

7. With one hand in each of the two superior quadrants, simultaneously display two fingers of one hand and one finger of the other. Ask the patient to identify the total number seen. Repeat step 7 to test the inferior quadrants.

8. If the patient cannot identify the fingers in one or more quadrants, record this as an abnormality.

9. Repeat steps 1 through 8 to test for the patient's left eye, with the patient's right eye covered.

Common Causes of Visual Field Abnormalities

☐ Tumors in the region of the optic chiasm

☐ Cerebral hemisphere tumors or strokes

☐ Retinal vascular occlusion

☐ Optic neuritis

☐ Ischemic optic neuropathy

☐ Glaucoma

Figure 1-5 Confrontation visual field test. The patient is instructed to identify the number of stationary fingers displayed well within the normal boundary of each field quadrant.

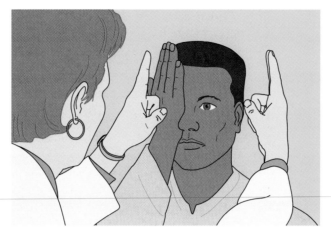

External Examination

The external eye examination screens for abnormalities of the ocular surface (cornea, conjunctiva) and surrounding tissues (eyelids, orbital structures). Corneal epithelial defects can be highlighted by staining the cornea with fluorescein dye.

Penlight Inspection

1. Under direct penlight illumination, inspect the eyelids and the skin of the face around the eye.
2. Separate the eyelids to examine the conjunctiva and cornea. Ask the patient to shift gaze direction to provide a more complete view.

Corneal Staining

1. Place a drop of topical anesthetic on the conjunctiva (see the Close-Up "Instillation of Medications in the Eye" in Chapter 7). Touch a wet fluorescein strip to the conjunctival cul-de-sac (Figure 1-6A).
2. With the ophthalmoscope set between +5 and +10 diopters or with a magnifying loupe, look for green patches or lines on the corneal surface that do not move after the patient blinks (Figure 1-6B). These defects in the corneal epithelium will stand out more clearly under cobalt-blue light.

Common Causes of External Eye Abnormalities

- Proptosis, or exophthalmos: Graves' disease, orbital inflammation, orbital tumor, postseptal cellulitis, blunt injury
- Ptosis: cranial nerve III palsy, Horner's syndrome, myasthenia gravis

- Swollen eyelids: chalazion, stye, dacryocystitis
- Eyelid lacerations
- Tearing: dacryocystitis, orbital inflammation, ocular foreign body, atopic allergy, Graves' disease
- Discharge: allergic, bacterial, viral, and chlamydial conjunctivitis, dacryocystitis, orbital inflammation
- Injected, swollen, or hemorrhagic conjunctiva: red eye disorders
- Corneal opacities and erosions: infectious and noninfectious keratitis, conjunctival and corneal foreign bodies

Pupillary Examination

The pupillary examination detects neurologic abnormalities that disturb the pupillary reflex arc, thereby altering the size of the pupils in dim light and their reactions to direct light. The three components to this examination comprise measuring pupil size in dim light (assesses the motor, or efferent, limb of the pupillary reflex arc); evaluating pupil response to direct light (assesses both the motor and the sensory, or afferent, limbs); and the swinging-light test (assesses only the sensory limb).

Pupil Size in Dim Light

Pupils that differ in size (anisocoria) by more than 1 mm in dim light may be clinically important. Because anisocoria can be obscured if the pupils are constricted, it is best to perform this procedure in the dimmest light possible.

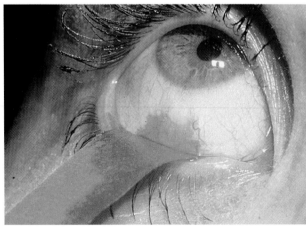

A

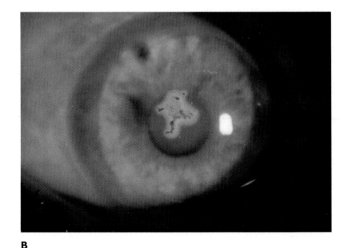

B

Figure 1-6 Corneal staining. (**A**) A moistened fluorescein strip is applied to the lower conjunctival cul-de-sac. (**B**) In cobalt-blue light, a green stain indicates a damaged corneal epithelium, in this case due to herpes simplex keratitis. (Part B courtesy W.K. Kellogg Eye Center, University of Michigan.)

1. Have the patient fixate on an object at least 10 feet away in a darkened room.

2. Position a penlight below the patient's eye to avoid fixation on the light, which would induce pupil constriction. Illuminate both eyes with the least amount of light necessary to discern pupil size.

3. Measure the pupil diameter in both eyes with a millimeter ruler or the pupil gauge generally found on the near vision card.

Pupil Response to Direct Light

1. Shine a penlight directly into the right eye.

2. Observe and record whether the pupil constricts strongly (rapidly and completely, or 3+ to 4+), weakly (slowly and incompletely, or 1+ to 2+), or not at all.

3. Repeat the test with the other eye.

Swinging-Light Test

1. In a darkened room with the patient fixating a distant target, shine the penlight directly into the right eye. Note the pupillary constriction.

2. Swing the penlight quickly over the bridge of the nose, shine it in the left eye, and observe the pupillary response. Normally, the pupil will either constrict slightly or remain at its previous size. An abnormal response is dilation of the pupil.

3. Swing the light back so that it shines in the right eye and observe the response. A normal response is either slight constriction or no change in size. Pupil dilation is an abnormal response.

4. Repeat these steps several times rhythmically until it is clear whether pupillary responses are normal or whether one pupil consistently dilates, termed a *relative afferent pupillary defect*. The eye with a relative afferent pupillary defect must have an optic nerve lesion or a severe retinal lesion.

Figure 1-7 summarizes the swinging-light test.

Common Causes of Pupillary Abnormalities

□ Anisocoria: benign idiopathic anisocoria (neither pupil is abnormal); cranial nerve III palsy (the larger pupil is abnormal, extraocular and levator muscle weakness is usually present); Horner's syndrome (the smaller pupil is abnormal); Adie's syndrome, ocular trauma or inflammation, prescription or over-the-counter eyedrops, Argyll Robertson (luetic) pupil (the larger or the smaller pupil may be abnormal)

□ Weak reaction to direct light: same causes as produce anisocoria (except Horner's syndrome), as well as optic nerve and retinal disease

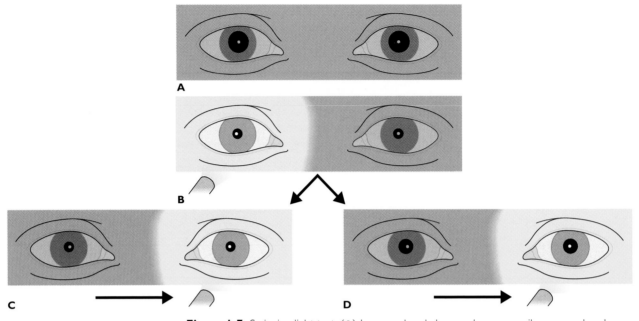

Figure 1-7 Swinging-light test. (**A**) In normal and abnormal cases, pupils are equal and unconstricted in dim illumination. (**B**) In the normal case, the right and left pupils constrict equally to light directed at the right eye; (**C**) there is no change in pupil size when light is quickly directed at the left eye. (**D**) In the abnormal case, both pupils dilate when light is quickly directed at the left eye. The left eye is said to display a relative afferent pupillary defect, probably because the optic nerve is damaged on that side.

- Relative afferent pupillary defect: optic neuritis, ischemic optic neuropathy, chiasmal area tumors, retinal artery or vein occlusion, retinal detachment, acute angle-closure glaucoma

Motility and Alignment Examination

This portion of the examination screens for abnormalities in eye movements and for ocular misalignment (strabismus). The three procedures include measurement of ocular movements, the corneal light reflection test, and the cover test. For all three, the examiner and patient are seated facing each other, about 10 to 14 inches apart.

Ocular Movements

1. Ask the patient to follow your finger or a penlight with the eyes as you move it from straight ahead to the far right and left, then up and down. Elevate the upper lid with your thumb to observe down gaze.

2. Note whether the amplitude of eye movements is normal or abnormal, defined as follows: In right and left gaze, the sclera should disappear into the canthus completely. In up gaze, half the cornea should disappear behind the upper eyelid. In down gaze, two thirds of the cornea should disappear behind the lower eyelid.

3. Note if an ocular oscillation (nystagmus) is present in any field of gaze.

4. Record amplitude of eye movements by scoring normal amplitude as 100% and lesser amplitudes accordingly.

5. Record nystagmus according to its presence in each field of gaze (eg, straight-ahead gaze, right gaze, left gaze, up gaze, and down gaze).

Corneal Light Reflection Test

This procedure compares the position of the corneal light reflection in both eyes (Figure 1-8). If the eyes are aligned, the light reflection appears symmetric in the two eyes. If the eyes are not aligned, one image will be displaced.

Figure 1-8 Corneal light reflection test. (**A**) Normal alignment: the light reflections are centered on both corneas. (**B**) Left esotropia: the light reflection is outwardly displaced on the left cornea. (**C**) Left exotropia: the light reflection is inwardly displaced on the left cornea. (**D**) Left hypertropia: the light reflection is downwardly displaced on the left cornea. (**E**) Right hypertropia: the light reflection is downwardly displaced on the right cornea.

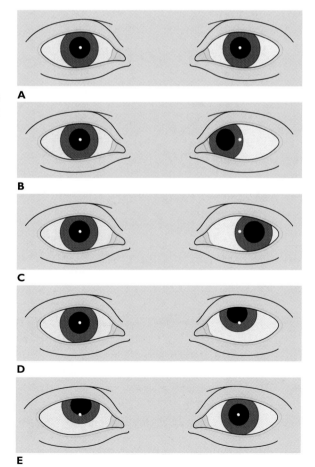

A

B

C

D

E

1. Have the patient fixate on a small target you hold adjacent to the penlight. Position the penlight at least 10 feet from the patient's eyes.

2. Shine the penlight onto both corneas simultaneously.

3. Compare the positions of the two corneal light reflections, and record the result as either normal or abnormal according to the list below.

Position of Reflections	Ocular Alignment
Symmetric	Normal
Outwardly displaced	Convergent misalignment (esotropia)
Inwardly displaced	Divergent misalignment (exotropia)
Downwardly or upwardly displaced	Vertical misalignment (hypertropia)

Cover Test

The cover test (Figure 1-9) is a more accurate test for ocular misalignment than is the corneal light reflection test, but it requires more cooperation from the patient and more skill on the part of the examiner. Parental help can be useful in testing children under 3 years of age.

1. Have the patient fixate on an eye chart or object 15 to 20 feet away. For children, use an attention-getting device, such as a toy, and, if necessary, have the parent encourage the child to look at the object.

Figure 1-9 Cover test. (**A**) Esotropia. (**1**) With the patient's gaze directed straight ahead, the corneal reflections indicate left esotropia. (**2**) When the right eye is occluded, the left eye moves outward to "pick up" fixation. (**B**) Exotropia. (**1**) With the patient's gaze directed straight ahead, the corneal reflections indicate left exotropia. (**2**) When the right eye is occluded, the left eye moves inward to "pick up" fixation.

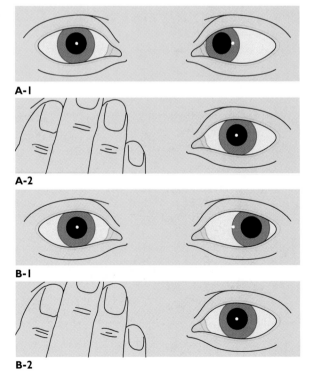

A-1

A-2

B-1

B-2

2. Cover the patient's right eye swiftly with your hand or an occluder, and observe the left eye for a fixational movement.

3. Uncover the right eye, swiftly cover the left eye, and observe the right eye for a fixational movement.

4. Record the status of alignment according to the list below.

Eye Movement	Ocular Alignment
None	Normal
Outward	Esotropia
Inward	Exotropia
Downward or upward	Hypertropia

Common Causes of Motility and Alignment Abnormalities

☐ Congenital and childhood-onset strabismus

☐ Cranial nerve palsies

☐ Orbital trauma

☐ Graves' disease

☐ Myasthenia gravis

☐ Stroke

☐ Brain tumor

Ophthalmoscopic Examination

The direct ophthalmoscope is used to evoke red reflexes and to view the retina and optic nerve.

Red Reflexes

The presence of normal red reflexes is an indication that the ocular media are free of opacities, that there is no large refractive error, and that the eyes are aligned (Figure 1-10).

Figure 1-10 Ophthalmoscopic examination of red reflexes. The relatively dull reflex from the patient's left eye is the result of a vitreous hemorrhage. (Courtesy W.K. Kellogg Eye Center, University of Michigan.)

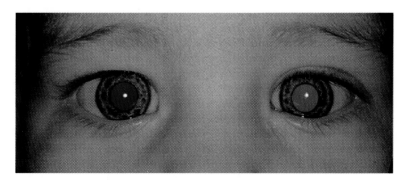

1. At a viewing distance of 1 foot, with the lens dioptric power setting on 0 (zero), shine the light through the pupils.

2. Compare the brightness of the red reflexes in the two eyes.

Retinal and Optic Nerve Examination

Direct ophthalmoscopic evaluation of the retina and optic nerve head is best performed with the patient's pupil pharmacologically dilated (see the Close-Up "Pupillary Dilation for Ophthalmoscopy"). Even through dilated pupils, however, direct ophthalmoscopy allows only a limited view of the retinal periphery and may fail to disclose important pathology, such as retinal detachment, which may be restricted to this region.

1. Using your right eye to examine the patient's right eye and your left to examine the patient's left, hold the direct ophthalmoscope 12 to 18 inches from the patient's face. Select the large-beam aperture and set the dioptric power at 0. Ask the patient to fixate on a distant target with both eyes. If the patient is unable to keep the eye open, elevate the upper lid with your thumb.

2. Approach the patient's eye gradually, dialing the ophthalmoscope's dioptric power until the optic fundus is in focus, aiming the beam first at the optic disc (15° medially), so as to cause minimal pupil constriction. If the pupil diameter is narrow, switch to the small lens aperture for a better view. To further improve the view, get as close to the patient's eye as possible.

3. Evaluate these features of the optic disc:

Feature	Normal	Abnormal
Color	Pink	White
Cup size	$<\frac{1}{2}$ disc radius	$>\frac{1}{2}$ disc radius
Margins	Flat, distinct	Raised, indistinct

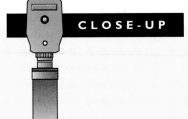

CLOSE-UP   **PUPILLARY DILATION FOR OPHTHALMOSCOPY**

The recommended mydriatic agent for ophthalmoscopic screening is phenylephrine 2.5% (2 drops instilled 1 minute apart). Although this sympathomimetic drug is weaker than the parasympatholytic drugs used by ophthalmologists (tropicamide, cyclopentolate), phenylephrine is a safe agent that stimulates the iris dilator, producing adequate mydriasis within 15 minutes and lasting only about 2 hours. The risk of angle-closure glaucoma is extremely low and there are no other important side effects to the diagnostic use of this mydriatic agent in a 2.5% strength.

4. Examine the retinal vessels from the disc outward to their second bifurcation, looking for these signs:
   □ Abnormal light reflections (silver-wiring)
   □ Arteriovenous nicking
   □ Vascular sheathing
   □ Intravascular yellow-white plaques
   □ Neovascularization
5. Examine the nonvascular parts of the retina for
   □ Hemorrhages (red)
   □ Cotton-wool spots (retinal microinfarcts)
   □ Hard exudates (extravascular proteolipid deposits)
6. Examine the macula for
   □ Drusen (discrete yellowish deposits in the deep retina)
   □ Gliosis (discrete white areas of repair)
   □ Hemorrhage (red)
   □ Infiltrate (nondiscrete white areas of inflammation)

Figure 1-11 summarizes the ophthalmoscopic examination.

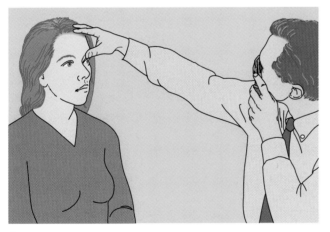

A

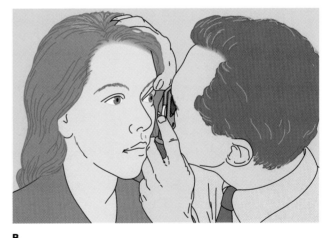

B

Figure 1-11 Ophthalmoscopic examination of the retina and optic nerve. (**A**) Set the dioptric power at 0, instruct the patient to fixate on the distant target, and elevate the patient's upper lid with your thumb. (**B**) Approach as close as possible to the eyelashes, aiming the beam 15° nasally toward the optic disc and dialing a dioptric power that places the optic nerve in best focus. (**C**) Starting at the blue arrowhead, follow a viewing path indicated by the arrows, noting features of the optic disc, retinal vessels, and posterior retina. (Part C courtesy W.K. Kellogg Eye Center, University of Michigan.)

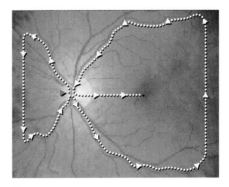

C

Common Causes of Ophthalmoscopic Abnormalities

- Absent or dull red reflex: corneal opacity, hyphema, cataract, vitreous hemorrhage, endophthalmitis, large refractive error, ocular misalignment
- Optic disc pallor: optic nerve disease
- Optic disc cupping: glaucoma
- Raised and indistinct optic disc margins: papilledema (increased intracranial pressure), optic neuritis, ischemic optic neuropathy
- Retinal arteriolar silver-wiring, arteriovenous nicking: long-standing systemic hypertension
- Retinal vascular sheathing: vasculitis and occlusive disease
- Retinal arterial plaque: retinal embolus from the heart or internal carotid artery
- Retinal hemorrhage: diabetes, hypertension, blood dyscrasia, ocular or head trauma, sudden increase in intracranial pressure, retinal vein occlusion
- Cotton-wool spots: hypertension, diabetes, connective tissue disease, blood dyscrasia, AIDS
- Hard exudates: diabetes, retinal vascular malformation
- Macular drusen, gliosis, hemorrhage: age-related macular degeneration
- Macular infiltrate: retinitis

CHAPTER 2

The Asymptomatic Patient

This chapter reviews the rationale, frequency, and components of the screening examination for the routine, periodic evaluation of patients without ophthalmic symptoms. Chapters 3, 4, and 5 present information helpful in evaluating and treating patients with ophthalmic symptoms and signs.

Rationale

Vision-threatening conditions can exist for some time without causing symptoms for several reasons:

☐ The visual deficit affects only one eye; the patient is unaware of visual loss because the unaffected eye compensates for the other eye.

☐ The visual deficit develops slowly or affects only the patient's peripheral vision, as in primary open-angle glaucoma.

☐ Damage is occurring but has not yet caused a visual deficit, as in uveal melanoma and diabetic retinopathy.

The ophthalmic screening of children is particularly critical for two reasons: children typically do not report symptoms, and the visual system within the first decade of life is quickly damaged by visual deprivation (eg, amblyopia). If such visual deprivation is discovered and relieved early enough, vision is rapidly recovered.

Frequency and Components of the Examination

The frequency of ophthalmic screening is based on age and estimated risk for disease. There are four risk groups: low-risk children, high-risk children, low-risk adults, and high-risk adults. The components of the screening examination (see Chapter 1) and their objectives are listed below for each age and risk group.

Low-Risk Children

Low-risk children are screened as neonates and at 6 months, 3 years, and 5 to 6 years of age. After age 6, individuals are screened according to adult standards.

Neonate

- □ External (penlight) examination for surface abnormalities of the eye and surrounding tissues
- □ Ocular alignment (corneal reflections)
- □ Ophthalmoscopy for red reflexes

Age 6 Months

- □ Ability to fix and follow light, face, or small toy
- □ External (penlight) examination for surface abnormalities of the eye and surrounding tissues
- □ Pupillary examination
- □ Ocular alignment (corneal reflections)
- □ Ophthalmoscopy for red reflexes

Age 3

- □ Visual acuity by picture chart or tumbling E chart
- □ External (penlight) examination for surface abnormalities of the eye and surrounding tissues
- □ Pupillary examination
- □ Ocular motility and alignment (ocular movements, cover test, and corneal reflections)
- □ Ophthalmoscopy for red reflexes and examination of retina and optic nerve

Age 5 to 6

- □ Visual acuity by Snellen method
- □ External (penlight) examination for surface abnormalities of the eye and surrounding tissues
- □ Pupillary examination

□ Ocular motility and alignment (ocular movements, cover test, and corneal reflections)

□ Ophthalmoscopy for red reflexes and examination of retina and optic nerve

High-Risk Children

High-risk children fall into four groups: (1) prematurity (birth weight less than 1250 g); (2) family history of congenital ocular abnormality (eg, cataract, retinoblastoma), strabismus or amblyopia; (3) maternal intrauterine or cervico-vaginal infection or substance abuse; (4) systemic condition with vision-threatening ocular manifestations.

Because a rapidly progressing condition may threaten the developing visual system, infants and children in these high-risk categories should be referred to an ophthalmologist as soon as the high-risk factor has been identified. A schedule of followup ophthalmic screening examinations and ophthalmologic examinations should then be arranged in concert with the ophthalmologist.

Low-Risk Adults

The scheduling of ophthalmic screening examinations of low-risk adults is divided into two age brackets: age 6 to 40, and over age 40.

Age 6 to 40

Visual acuity measurement every 3 years is recommended. Because of the extremely low prevalence of ocular disease in this age group, more extensive ophthalmic screening is generally limited to patients with ophthalmic symptoms. Referral to an ophthalmologist is indicated only if an abnormality has been detected or the patient has ophthalmic symptoms.

Over Age 40

A complete screening examination every 2 years is recommended. Patients in this age group also require examinations by an ophthalmologist every 2 to 4 years to provide optical correction for presbyopia and to monitor for glaucoma. Screening for glaucoma by tonometry was formerly considered an important task for general physicians, but a tonometric reading alone is of limited value. Tonometry is more meaningful if performed as part of a more comprehensive ophthalmologic assessment, including evaluation of the optic disc.

High-Risk Adults

High-risk adults fall into five groups: (1) personal history of retinal detachment, serious ocular trauma, or persistent visual loss in one or both eyes; (2) personal history of diabetes (see the Close-Up), hypertension, or sickle cell disease; (3) family history of glaucoma or other heritable ocular disease;

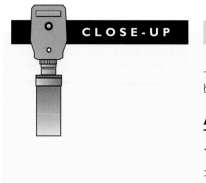

INITIAL OPHTHALMOLOGIC EXAM OF DIABETIC PATIENTS

The recommended timing of initial ophthalmologic examination of diabetic patients is based on the prevalence of treatable retinopathy established in population studies.

Age at Diagnosis	First Ophthalmologic Examination
<30 years old	5 years after diagnosis
>30 years old	At the time of diagnosis

(4) African-Americans, because the risk of glaucoma is three times greater than that for whites; (5) over age 65.

A complete screening examination every 1 to 2 years is recommended. Such patients also require evaluation by an ophthalmologist shortly after the high-risk factor has been identified. The schedule of periodic followup ophthalmologic evaluations should be determined by the ophthalmologist.

CHAPTER 3

Common Symptoms and Signs

The successful evaluation of common ophthalmic symptoms and signs depends on appropriate history-taking and ophthalmic screening. This chapter describes the management of 13 common ophthalmic complaints, with the most serious and emergent entities presented first. Specific history-taking questions and components of the examination, together with management and referral suggestions, are presented for each complaint. The red eye is covered separately in Chapter 4 because it has so many diagnostic possibilities. Chapter 5 discusses the common presentations of ophthalmic trauma.

Acute Persistent Visual Loss

Acute visual loss that persists beyond 1 hour requires emergent treatment. The differential diagnosis includes keratitis, acute glaucoma, endophthalmitis, vitreous or retinal hemorrhage, retinal detachment, acute maculopathy, retinal artery occlusion, retinal vein occlusion, optic neuritis, ischemic optic neuropathy, occipital (visual) cortex infarction, and a psychogenic disturbance. Table 3-1, "Acute Persistent Visual Loss," compares symptoms, signs, and urgency of treatment for these conditions.

Emergent = immediately. Urgent = within 48 hours. Nonurgent = later than 48 hours.

TABLE 3-1
Acute Persistent Visual Loss

	Pain	Red Eye	Afferent Pupil Defect	Ophthal-moscopic Findings	Urgency of Treatment	Comments
Keratitis	+	+	−	−	Emergent	Early treatment may avert damage to subepithelial tissues that leads to permanent visual loss.
Acute angle-closure glaucoma	+	+	+/−	−	Emergent	Diagnosis depends on accurate measurement of intraocular pressure. If emergent referral is impossible, make a presumptive diagnosis and administer pressure-lowering agents immediately.
Endophthalmitis	+	+/−	−	↓ Red reflex	Emergent	Infection of the intraocular tissues caused by surface pathogens or blood-borne sepsis. Emergent anti-infective treatment by parenteral and intravitreal routes is necessary to preserve vision.
Retinal or vitreous hemorrhage	−	−	−	↓ Red reflex (if vitreous hemorrhage is extensive)	Urgent	Caused by rupture of retinal vessels in hypertension, diabetes, arteriosclerosis, sickle cell disease, other blood dyscrasias, and as a consequence of retinal tearing. Urgency of referral is mainly to rule out retinal tear and detachment and to control blood pressure.
Retinal detachment	−	−	+/−	Retinal separation	Emergent	Difficult to diagnose without indirect ophthalmoscope and other specialized instruments. To preserve visual acuity, reattachment surgery must be performed before the macular portion of retina detaches.
Acute maculopathy	−	−	−	Altered color in macula*	Urgent	Caused by subretinal hemorrhage, retinal tear, edema from leaky blood vessels, and inflammation. Although a color change is usually apparent, the affected area is small and poorly seen unless viewed through specialized lenses and pharmacologically dilated pupils. Urgent laser treatment sometimes is indicated to prevent further subretinal hemorrhage.

* Red = hemorrhage; white = infiltration, inflammation.

TABLE 3-1 (continued)
Acute Persistent Visual Loss

	Pain	Red Eye	Afferent Pupil Defect	Ophthal-moscopic Findings	Urgency of Treatment	Comments
Retinal artery occlusion	–	–	+	Cherry-red spot	Emergent	Caused most often by thrombosis or embolism. The ischemic retina appears turbid, but is often difficult to recognize unless the pupils are pharmacologically dilated. If the macula is involved, a cherry-red spot will be centered there. Intraocular pressure is lowered immediately in hopes of promoting blood flow.
Retinal vein occlusion	–	–	+/–	Retinal hemorrhage	Urgent	Caused by thrombosis. The retinal surface appears blood-splattered. There is no urgency in treatment, but urgency of referral is based on difficulty of diagnosis.
Optic neuritis	+	–	+	+/– Swollen disc	Urgent	Usually caused by acute demyelination. Intravenous corticosteroid treatment within 8 days does not affect vision but restrains development of other neurologic manifestations.
Ischemic optic neuropathy	–	–	+	Swollen disc	Emergent[†]	Usually caused by arteriosclerotic occlusion of small arterioles, for which there is no immediate treatment. In patients over 60 years old, must rule out cranial (temporal) arteritis, for which high-dose corticosteroid treatment is emergent to prevent further visual loss.
Occipital (visual) cortex infarction	–	–	–	–	Urgent	Caused by embolism or thrombosis in vertebrobasilar circulation. Often limited to one hemifield, but may impair visual acuity in both eyes if bilateral. Often no other neurologic manifestations, at least initially. Urgency of referral is based on the possibility of evolving brainstem stroke.
Psychogenic disturbance	+/–	–	–	–	Nonurgent	Patient is consciously or unconsciously dissembling. Rule out organic causes first, which may be difficult.

[†] Arteritic type only.

History-Taking

- **How long ago did the visual loss take place?**
  The more recent, the more urgent.

- **How suddenly did it happen?**
  Suddenness suggests ischemia, hemorrhage, or compression.

- **Has it worsened, improved, or remained unchanged?**
  Worsening conditions are more urgent.

- **Has it affected one eye or both?**
  Binocular involvement suggests a cerebral lesion.

- **Has it happened before?**
  Previous occurrence reduces urgency.

- **Was the lost sight confined to a particular area of visual space?**
  If so, a retinal, optic nerve, or cerebral lesion is likely.

- **Was there pain around the eye?**
  If so, consider an anterior ocular cause or optic neuritis.

- **Did nausea and vomiting accompany the ocular pain?**
  Suggests acute angle-closure glaucoma.

- **Has there been a sudden cluster of new flashes or floaters?**
  Suggests vitreous hemorrhage or retinal detachment.

- **Has the patient had an ophthalmic disease, trauma, or surgery?**
  Suggests an ocular cause.

- **Has there been a recent change in systemic medications?**
  Medications can cause visual loss.

Examination

- External examination: look for circumcorneal injection, or ciliary flush, with diffuse corneal haze (acute glaucoma) or corneal opacities (keratitis); stain the cornea with fluorescein if keratitis is suspected

- Confrontation visual fields: look particularly for a homonymous hemi-anopia (cerebral lesion)

- Pupillary examination: look for a middilated unreactive pupil (acute glaucoma) or a relative afferent pupillary defect (optic nerve or retinal lesion, retinal artery occlusion, and sometimes acute glaucoma and retinal vein occlusion)

- Ophthalmoscopic examination: note an absent red reflex (endophthalmitis, vitreous hemorrhage), a cherry-red spot (central retinal artery occlusion), retinal surface blood (hypertension, dyscrasia, retinal vein occlusion), retinal separation (detachment), or optic nerve head swelling (ischemic optic neuropathy, optic neuritis)

Treatment and Referral

☐ Institute emergency treatment for the following three conditions and refer emergently:

1. Central retinal artery occlusion: Massage the globe with the index fingers of each hand (5 seconds pressure, 5 seconds release) 20 times to reduce the intraocular pressure. The low pressure may move an embolus or reopen a thrombosed retinal artery. An alternative treatment used to lower pressure is acetazolamide 500 mg administered intravenously; rebreathing CO_2 and taking nifedipine sublingually may be used to promote ocular blood flow.

2. Acute angle-closure glaucoma: Instill topical pilocarpine 2% every 5 minutes for three doses, topical timolol 0.5% one dose, and acetazolamide 500 mg one dose by mouth or vein.

3. Ischemic optic neuropathy (optic nerve infarction) in giant-cell arteritis: Immediately commence prednisone 2 mg/kg/day orally or methylprednisolone 250 mg every 6 hours intravenously.

☐ Refer emergently patients with keratitis, endophthalmitis, or retinal detachment.

☐ Refer all other conditions urgently.

Anisocoria

Anisocoria is a difference in the size of the pupils in the dimmest illumination needed to examine the pupils. Anisocoria is considered potentially pathologic if it is greater than 1 mm. Neurogenic causes include cranial nerve III palsy, Horner's syndrome, Adie's syndrome, Argyll Robertson (luetic) pupil, ocular trauma or inflammation, eyedrops, and benign idiopathic anisocoria. Myogenic causes include congenital malformation, inflammation, and trauma of the iris.

History-Taking

☐ **When was the anisocoria first noted?**
The more recent, the more urgent.

☐ **Does the patient report ptosis or diplopia?**
Suggests more widespread neurologic disturbance.

☐ **Has there been trauma or eye surgery?**
Common cause of iris sphincter damage.

Examination

☐ External examination: note whether ptosis is present (cranial nerve III lesion or Horner's syndrome)

- Pupillary examination: document the presence of anisocoria by measuring pupil size in dim light; test the reactions to direct light (Horner's syndrome has normal pupil reactions)
- Motility and alignment examination: Measure ocular movements (weakness suggests a cranial nerve III palsy)

Treatment and Referral

- Refer urgently if a motility deficit or ptosis is present.
- Refer nonurgently if anisocoria is isolated.

Chronic Progressive Visual Loss

Chronic progressive visual loss may be due to refractive errors, to disturbances of clarity in the ocular media (cornea, lens, vitreous), or to lesions of the neural visual pathway from the retina to the visual cortex. In some patients, it is psychogenic.

History-Taking

- **Does the visual loss affect one eye or both?**
  Refractive problems are usually binocular.
- **Does the visual loss affect distance or near vision, or both?**
  If one or the other—but not both—may be a refractive cause.
- **Does the visual loss affect a portion of the visual field?**
  Suggests a retinal or other neural cause.
- **Can vision be improved by squinting?**
  Suggests a refractive cause.
- **When did the patient last have an ophthalmologic examination with normal results?**
  Establishes a baseline for the probable onset of the condition.

Examination

- External examination: look for corneal opacities (keratitis)
- Confrontation visual fields: look for any visual field defect (optic nerve, retinal, or cerebral lesion)
- Pupillary examination: look for a relative afferent pupillary defect (optic nerve or retinal lesion)
- Ophthalmoscopic examination: note an absent red reflex (cataract), optic disc pallor (optic nerve lesion), or macular drusen (age-related macular degeneration)

Treatment and Referral

☐ Refer keratitis emergently.

☐ Refer nonurgently patients with all other findings, as well as patients whose ophthalmic screening examination uncovers no abnormalities.

Diplopia

Diplopia, or double vision, can be either binocular or monocular. In the binocular form, the second image disappears when either eye is covered. The cause of binocular diplopia is always misalignment of the eyes, with one eye fixating on the target and the other seeing it as displaced.

In monocular diplopia, double vision persists even when one eye is covered. In contrast to the binocular variant, monocular diplopia is generated either by cataract or by uncorrected refractive error. In monocular diplopia, the second image often appears slightly superimposed on the first image ("ghosting").

History-Taking

☐ **Is the diplopia eliminated by covering either eye?**
Suggests ocular misalignment, or strabismus.

☐ **Were the two images separated or did they overlap?**
Separated: ocular misalignment. Overlapped: probably refractive error, or cataract.

☐ **If the two images were separated, was the separation in a horizontal, vertical, or oblique plane?**
Helps identify the orientation of the misalignment.

☐ **Is the diplopia present at all times and in all viewing directions?**
If so, misalignment should be readily found.

☐ **How long has the diplopia been present, and has the image separation increased, decreased, or remained the same?**
Helps define the course of the condition.

☐ **Has there been facial or severe head trauma?**
Helps localize the lesion to the orbit or the cranium.

☐ **Has there been periocular pain or headache?**
Suggests an intracranial inflammatory or neoplastic process.

Examination

☐ External examination: check for proptosis (orbital or periorbital lesion), ptosis (orbital or neural lesion), and ocular adnexal swelling (orbital or facial inflammation)

- ❑ Motility and alignment examination: confirm whether diplopia is monocular (uncorrected refractive error, cataract) or binocular (ocular misalignment) by asking the patient if the second image disappears as either eye is covered; test ocular movements and assess misalignment (corneal reflections and cover test) attributable to weakness of one or more of cranial nerves III, IV, and VI, restriction of eye movement (Graves' disease, orbital tumor, fracture), or myasthenia gravis
- ❑ Pupillary examination: look for anisocoria (suggesting neurologic disturbance)

Treatment and Referral

- ❑ Refer urgently to an ophthalmologist or a neurologist if the diplopia is binocular, of recent onset, and persistent.
- ❑ Refer nonurgently to an ophthalmologist if the diplopia is monocular. Monocular diplopia is nearly always due to a disturbance of the eye's refracting elements.

Distorted Vision

Distorted vision, or metamorphopsia, may be monocular and persistent or binocular and transient. In monocular and persistent distorted vision, images in the center of the visual field appear smaller or warped (Figure 3-1). The symptom is caused by edema or scarring of the macular photoreceptors (retinal metamorphopsia) secondary to a variety of retinal diseases—most commonly, age-related macular degeneration. Binocular and transient distorted vision may (rarely) arise in patients suffering seizures secondary to stroke, tumor, or inflammation of the posterior cerebral hemispheres (cerebral metamorphopsia). Images often appear grotesquely distorted in all parts of the field of vision.

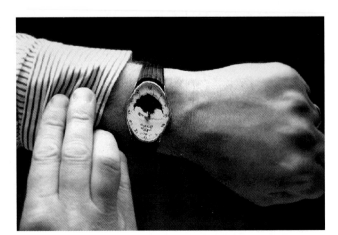

Figure 3-1 Retinal metamorphopsia. The image is distorted at the area of fixation. (Reproduced with permission from Burde RM, Savino PJ, Trobe JD: *Clinical Decisions in Neuro-Ophthalmology.* 2nd ed. St Louis: Mosby–Year Book; 1992.)

History-Taking

☐ **What was the shape of the distorted images?**
A curved and minified image suggests a retinal lesion.

☐ **Was the distortion confined to one eye?**
Suggests a retinal lesion.

☐ **Has there been recent ocular disease, trauma, or surgery?**
May contribute to a retinal cause.

☐ **Has there been recent cerebral disease, trauma, or surgery?**
May contribute to a cerebral cause.

☐ **Are there other manifestations of seizures?**
Suggests a cerebral cause.

Examination

☐ Visual acuity: ask the patient if letters appear distorted or smaller or if straight lines (on a sheet of paper or on the wall) appear curved or crooked (suggests retinal metamorphopsia)

☐ Confrontation visual fields: look for a homonymous hemianopia (suggests cerebral metamorphopsia)

☐ Ophthalmoscopic examination: look for drusen, hemorrhage, gliosis, or infiltration of the macula

Treatment and Referral

☐ For retinal metamorphopsia, refer urgently to an ophthalmologist because delay may render subretinal new blood vessels untreatable by laser.

☐ For cerebral metamorphopsia, refer urgently to a neurologist because of the possibility of stroke, seizure, or tumor.

Fading Vision

Patients often report that images disappear from view after prolonged viewing, especially reading. This symptom is usually psychogenic and should be distinguished from abrupt transient visual loss (see "Transient Visual Loss").

History-Taking

☐ **Did images fade slowly or abruptly?**
Slow fade is psychogenic.

☐ **Was it provoked by sustained reading or other types of viewing activities?**
Suggests psychogenic.

☐ **Was it provoked by assuming the upright posture?**
Suggests papilledema.

Examination

☐ Perform a complete ophthalmic screening examination, expecting the results to be negative but ruling out swollen discs if the symptom is brought on by standing.

Treatment and Referral

☐ Reassure the patient; refer nonurgently if the diagnosis is in doubt.

Flashes

Flashes of light are caused by inappropriate firing of neuronal elements within the visual pathway. Although any part of the visual pathway may generate flashes of light, the two most common sources are the retina and the visual cortex.

Retinal flashes are associated with a partially detached vitreous body, which, by tugging on the retina, causes the photoreceptors to fire. Because the vitreous detachment may progress to a retinal detachment, the new onset or a sudden worsening of flashes is a basis for urgent ophthalmologic referral. Retinal flashes are usually brief, confined to the peripheral visual field, and provoked by eye or head movement or trauma. They are especially common in the elderly, patients who have had intraocular surgery, and individuals with high myopia.

Cortical flashes have two underlying causes: migraine and occipital epilepsy. Often called *scintillations*, they tend to last longer and have more geometric shapes than retinal flashes. In migraine, the scintillations are often zigzag, are similar from episode to episode, and generally progress across the visual field over a standard time interval of 20 to 30 minutes (Figure 3-2). Headache may or may not follow the scintillations. The scintillations of occipital epilepsy lack a characteristic shape, are variable between episodes, and do not march across the visual field. Headache may be present but does not necessarily occur with the scintillations.

History-Taking

☐ **Did the flashes march across the visual field?**
Migraine: march across field. Epilepsy: stationary.

☐ **Were the flashes provoked by eye or head movement?**
If so, the origin is probably retinal.

☐ **How long did the flashes last?**
Retinal: seconds. Migraine or epilepsy: minutes.

☐ **Has there been an increase in floaters or new visual loss?**
Floaters suggest a retinal cause; new visual loss needs further definition.

☐ **Has there been recent head or eye trauma or eye surgery?**
Suggests a retinal cause.

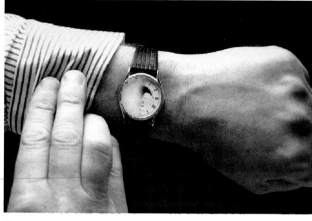

A

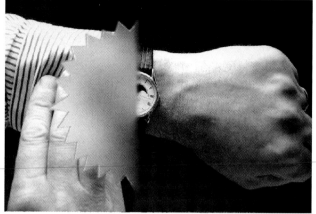

B

Figure 3-2 Typical scintillations of migraine. (**A**) A small scotoma with jagged edges ("fortifications") is seen by both eyes to the left of fixation. (**B**) After 10 minutes, the scotoma covers half of the left visual field. (**C**) After 20 minutes, the entire left visual field is obscured and headache begins. The jagged edges and progressive enlargement of the scotoma are common but not necessary features of migraine. (Reproduced with permission from Burde RM, Savino PJ, Trobe JD: *Clinical Decisions in Neuro-Ophthalmology.* 2nd ed. St Louis: Mosby–Year Book; 1992.)

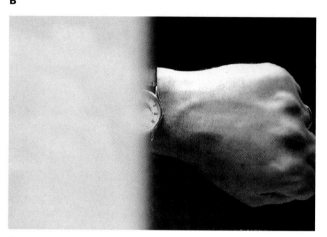

C

□ **Was headache present and, if so, what was its timing in relation to the flashes?**
Migraine has stereotypic features; try to elicit them.

Examination

□ Visual acuity examination: look for subnormal vision (retinal detachment)

□ Confrontation visual fields: look for a monocular visual field defect (retinal detachment) or a binocular defect (visual cortex lesion)

□ Pupillary examination: look for a relative afferent pupillary defect (retinal detachment)

□ Ophthalmoscopic examination: note an absent red reflex (vitreous hemorrhage), retinal separation (detachment)

Treatment and Referral

☐ Refer an observed retinal detachment emergently.

☐ Refer urgently a first occurrence or a sudden, marked worsening of retinal flashes to rule out retinal detachment. Refer emergently if the flashes are combined with acute visual acuity or field loss.

☐ If the flashes are chronically recurrent and unchanged, refer to rule out retinal detachment only if flashes increase in frequency or intensity.

☐ Treat the headache component if the flashes seem to be consistent with migraine.

☐ Refer nonurgently for neurologic evaluation if occipital epilepsy cannot be excluded.

Floaters

Floaters are described by patients as gray-black globs drifting in the visual field, typically lagging behind an eye movement. Occurring in one or both eyes and best seen against a white wall or a blue sky, they are solid aggregates that accumulate in the vitreous cavity as a degenerative result of aging. As such, they are predominantly a complaint of the elderly, although young and middle-aged myopic patients, who may have premature aging of the vitreous, also report having them. Floaters must be distinguished from blind spots, or scotomas, which do not drift in the field of vision or lag behind an eye movement.

Although floaters are usually benign, a rapid increase in their number is cause for further investigation. In such a situation, floaters may reflect a vitreous detachment or a retinal tear or detachment, especially in patients who have a family history of retinal detachment or a personal history of ocular trauma, inflammation, or surgery. Alternatively, floaters may be an indication of vitreous inflammation or hemorrhage, the latter associated with diabetes, hypertension, and sickle cell disease.

History-Taking

☐ **Did the patient report black globs that float or blank (blind) spots that are fixed?**
Vitreous floaters are usually not fixed; they lag behind an eye movement.

☐ **Has there been a sudden increase in floaters?**
Concern is retinal detachment.

☐ **Have there been flashes or new visual loss?**
Concern is retinal detachment.

☐ **Has there been recent eye or head trauma or eye surgery?**
Concern is retinal detachment.

☐ **Does the patient have a history of diabetes, hypertension, or sickle cell disease?**
Conditions associated with vitreous hemorrhage.

Examination

☐ Perform an ophthalmic screening examination as for flashes of light.

Treatment and Referral

☐ Refer urgently patients with ocular risk factors for vitreous hemorrhage or retinal detachment, those who have had ophthalmologic examinations with abnormal results, and those who have had a recent increase in floaters or flashes. Refer emergently if the floaters are accompanied by acute visual acuity or field loss.

☐ Reassure patients who do not fulfill these criteria that floaters are a benign symptom of the aging process.

Ocular Pain

Ocular pain may result from stimulation of trigeminal nerve fibers anywhere within the eye, the surrounding tissues, the deep orbit, and the base of the middle and anterior cranial fossae.

If the pain arises from the eye itself, external examination will sometimes reveal signs of inflammation—in other words, a red eye. Pain that comes from a corneal epithelial defect feels as if a grain of sand were in the eye (foreign-body sensation). If the pain arises from the eye's surrounding tissues, some evidence of eyelid swelling should be evident. However, deep and retro-orbital processes causing pain may produce no external evidence. The examiner should look for impairment of cranial nerve III, IV, or VI and for a Horner's syndrome—signs of a cavernous sinus lesion.

History-Taking

☐ **Is the pain constant or episodic? If episodic, what brings it on?**
If viewing tasks precipitate the pain, consider a refractive cause.

☐ **Does it feel like a grain of sand (foreign-body sensation)?**
Suggests a corneal epithelial defect.

☐ **Is it accompanied by joint or muscle stiffness, jaw claudication, visual loss, diplopia, proptosis, or ptosis?**
If so, consider giant-cell (temporal) arteritis, orbital or cavernous sinus syndrome. Pain accompanied by joint or muscle stiffness, jaw claudication, and visual loss suggests a diagnosis of giant-cell arteritis. Pain with proptosis, diplopia, ptosis, and visual loss points to orbital or cavernous sinus syndrome.

☐ **Has there been recent eye surgery, disease, or trauma?**
Suggests an ocular cause.

Examination

☐ Visual acuity examination: subnormal acuity suggests an ocular or neural cause

☐ Confrontation visual fields: any defect suggests a visual pathway lesion

☐ External examination: look for conjunctival hyperemia (keratitis, uveitis, scleritis, endophthalmitis, acute angle-closure glaucoma), ptosis (cranial nerve III palsy), proptosis (Graves' disease, orbital inflammation or tumor); if there are signs of keratitis, stain with fluorescein

☐ Pupillary examination: look for a relative afferent pupillary defect (optic neuritis)

☐ Motility and alignment examination: look for reduced eye movements (Graves' disease, other orbital inflammation, orbital tumor, cranial nerve III, IV, or VI palsy)

☐ Ophthalmoscopic examination: look for reduced red reflexes (keratitis, endophthalmitis), swelling of the optic disc (optic neuritis)

Treatment and Referral

☐ Refer urgently if ocular pain is accompanied by visual loss, diplopia, ptosis, or proptosis.

☐ Refer ocular pain alone nonurgently.

Proptosis

Proptosis, or exophthalmos, is forward displacement of the globe within the orbit, owing to an increase in orbital soft tissue or bone (Figure 3-3). The most common causes are Graves' disease, other orbital inflammations, and orbital tumor. **Caution:** Prominence of the globe caused by its enlargement or by lid retraction can be misinterpreted as proptosis.

History-Taking

☐ **How recent was the onset of the proptosis?**
The more recent, the more urgent.

☐ **Is there a history of hyperthyroidism or hypothyroidism?**
Graves' disease is associated with either one.

☐ **Does the patient have periocular pain?**
Severe pain is uncommon in Graves' disease; suggests an inflammation or tumor.

Figure 3-3 Proptosis. The right eye is displaced forward and downward by a sarcoma of the orbit. (Courtesy W.K. Kellogg Eye Center, University of Michigan.)

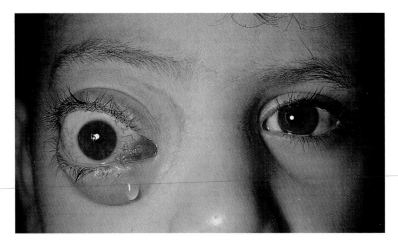

- [ ] **Is there lid retraction or lid lag?**
  Signs of Graves' disease.

- [ ] **Are the symptoms strictly monocular?**
  Graves' disease is usually binocular, although often asymmetric.

Examination

- [ ] Visual acuity: if subnormal, assume that the optic nerve or the globe is being deformed

- [ ] External examination: look for features that suggest Graves' disease (lid retraction and swelling, conjunctival hyperemia)

- [ ] Motility and alignment examination: reduced eye movement suggests considerable extraocular muscle swelling that may threaten optic nerve function

Treatment and Referral

- [ ] Refer urgently proptosis accompanied by visual loss, ocular misalignment, or motility disturbances.

- [ ] Refer proptosis alone nonurgently.

Ptosis

Ptosis, or blepharoptosis, is drooping of the upper eyelid. It may be caused by neurogenic or myogenic conditions. Neurogenic conditions may damage the parasympathetic (cranial nerve III) supply to the levator palpebrae superioris

Figure 3-4 Horner's syndrome. Ptosis of the left upper lid and miosis. The pupils react normally to direct light, and the eye movements are normal. The patient has an apical lung (Pancoast's) tumor.

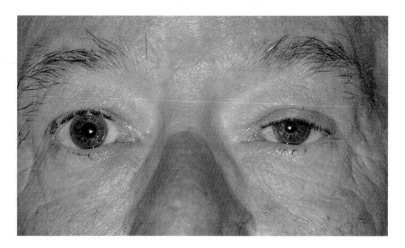

muscle, the sympathetic supply to Muller's muscle (Horner's syndrome, Figure 3-4), or the neuromuscular junction (myasthenia gravis). Myogenic conditions include congenital dystrophies of the levator muscle, senescent stretching and weakening of the levator tendon, inflammation, and trauma.

History-Taking

☐ **When did the ptosis begin?**
The more recent, the more urgent.

☐ **Has there been trauma to the eyes or neck?**
Eyelid trauma could be responsible. Neck trauma may cause a Horner's syndrome.

☐ **Does the patient have diplopia?**
Suggests the ptosis is part of a more widespread neurologic disturbance.

☐ **Does the patient have other symptoms that are compatible with myasthenia gravis?**
Myasthenia gravis is a frequently overlooked cause of ptosis.

Examination

☐ External examination: document the presence and severity of unilateral or bilateral ptosis (Horner's syndrome does not cause severe ptosis)

☐ Motility and alignment examination: look for associated ocular motility abnormalities; determine if they conform to a cranial nerve III, IV, or VI palsy

☐ Pupillary examination: look for anisocoria and reduced reaction to direct light (pupillary abnormalities are not found in myasthenia gravis; with ptosis, they suggest either Horner's syndrome or cranial nerve III palsy)

Figure 3-5 Entropion. Causes tearing, foreign-body sensation, and photophobia as the lashes of the lower lid rub against the corneal surface. Surgical repositioning of the lid is indicated. (Courtesy W.K. Kellogg Eye Center, University of Michigan.)

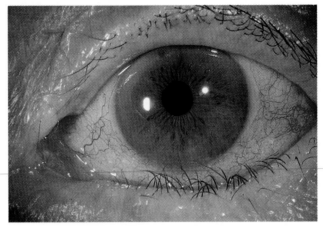

Treatment and Referral

☐ Refer urgently if either ocular motility defects or pupillary abnormalities are present.

☐ Refer nonurgently if ptosis is the only finding.

Tearing

Many people shed tears on cold, windy days. Otherwise, tearing is pathologic, and results either from overproduction or from poor drainage. Overproduction is usually caused by inflammation of the cornea, conjunctiva, or eyelids (Figure 3-5). Poor drainage is caused by poor apposition of the lower eyelid to the globe (eyelid deformity) or obstruction within the lacrimal drainage system (congenital nasolacrimal duct stenosis, inflammation, trauma, tumor).

Curiously, many people, including those with keratitis sicca, complain of tearing when they do not have enough tears. This is because baseline tear secretion may be deficient, causing corneal epithelial damage, which, in turn, stimulates reflex tearing.

History-Taking

☐ **Is the tearing of recent onset?**
Recent onset suggests a more urgent condition.

☐ **Is there ocular pain, photophobia, itching, or redness?**
Suggests an ocular inflammation.

☐ **Has there been trauma to the face or nose?**
Suggests a traumatic nasolacrimal obstruction.

☐ **Has there been a facial (Bell's) palsy?**
Suggests poor lid apposition to the globe.

☐ **Is there tenderness over the lacrimal sac area, and discharge from it?**
Suggests an infection.

☐ **Is there a complaint of dry mouth or arthritis?**
Suggests keratitis sicca.

Examination

☐ External examination: check for signs of poor lid apposition to the globe (entropion, ectropion, cranial nerve VII palsy), ocular inflammation; press on the lacrimal sac, attempting to elicit pain or discharge (dacryocystitis)

Treatment and Referral

☐ For infants under 6 months old, assume a delayed opening of the distal nasolacrimal duct.
1. Recommend daily massage by finger over the lacrimal sac in the direction of the nose.
2. Prescribe broad-spectrum topical antibiotics if a purulent discharge develops.
3. Refer for surgical probing if the signs persist beyond 9 months of age or if the lacrimal sac becomes distended or inflamed.

☐ Do not treat adults. Instead, refer under the following circumstances:
1. If tearing is a new symptom
2. If tearing is a manifestation of a deformity
3. If you suspect keratitis sicca or some other worrisome inflammation
4. If tearing is worsening or intolerable

Transient Visual Loss

Transient visual loss is defined as visual loss affecting one or both eyes that persists less than 1 day. Most often it lasts seconds to minutes and usually reflects migraine or temporary ischemia to the eye or visual cortex. The evaluation is largely directed at distinguishing between migraine and ischemia and at differentiating between local and remote causes of ocular ischemia.

History-Taking

☐ **How long did the visual loss last?**
Ischemia lasts seconds to minutes; migraine lasts much longer—20 minutes or more.

☐ **Has it happened before?**
Description of prior episodes may be differentially helpful.

☐ **Were there precipitating circumstances?**
Ischemia may be postural.

☐ **Did it affect one or both eyes?**
Migraine is usually binocular, but patients may not realize that.

☐ **Was the visual loss confined to an area of visual space?**
Hemianopic suggests an occipital locus; altitudinal suggests a retinal locus.

☐ **Did the patient also experience scintillations or headache?**
Scintillations suggest migraine, but not absolutely (see "Flashes"). Headache suggests migraine if it follows scintillations.

☐ **Was there imbalance, numbness, weakness, double vision, slurred speech, or difficulty in swallowing?**
Helps differentiate ischemia from migraine.

☐ **Is there a history of ocular disease, trauma, or surgery?**
May predispose to ocular causes of transient visual loss.

☐ **Has there been a recent change in medications?**
Systemic medications, such as agents for lowering blood pressure, may be causative.

☐ **Does the patient take oral contraceptives?**
Predisposes to migraine and thromboembolism.

☐ **Is there a history of transient ischemic cerebral attacks?**
Helps establish a predisposition.

☐ **Does the patient have arteriosclerotic risk factors?**
Most common setting for thromboembolic transient visual loss.

Examination

☐ Ophthalmoscopic examination: look for cotton-wool spots (patches of retinal whitening, a sign of microinfarct) and Hollenhorst plaques (intra-arterial retinal yellow-white spots, a sign of emboli; Figure 3-6)

Figure 3-6 Hollenhorst plaque causing transient visual loss. The yellow-white plug at the arterial bifurcation is evidence of a cholesterol-fibrin embolus originating in the proximal arterial tree, probably at the cervical-carotid bifurcation.

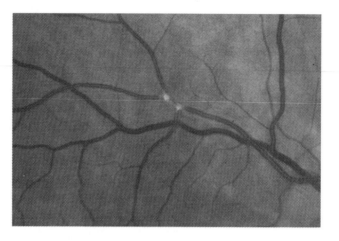

Treatment and Referral

☐ Treat a suspected transient ischemic attack with aspirin until further diagnostic workup is completed.

☐ Treat migraine if necessary.

☐ Refer nonurgently for detailed evaluation.

CHAPTER 4

The Red Eye

The red eye is an eye with conjunctival vascular congestion. This chapter defines 22 important red eye conditions, listing the main features of clinical presentation, followed by treatment and referral guidelines.

Some red eye conditions present a potential threat to vision. Because they usually require prompt and specialized care, these entities must be differentiated from the less threatening conditions, using the decision tree presented in Figure 4-1. (The numbers preceding the entities listed in the decision tree correspond to the numbers preceding the entities in the chapter.) The Close-Up "Features of a Dangerous Red Eye" on page 45 presents a quick reference list of symptoms and signs that accompany the serious conditions.

1: Chronic Blepharitis

Chronic blepharitis (Figure 4-2) is an inflammation of the lids that has two forms: (1) anterior, most often caused by *Staphylococcus aureus* infection of the skin, cilia follicles, or accessory glands of the eyelids; (2) posterior, infection or inflammation of the meibomian sebaceous glands.

The signs of blepharitis are difficult to recognize without magnification. Although the slit lamp provides the best view, the direct ophthalmoscope is a reasonable substitute. The eyelid inflammation produces a red eye by secondarily

---

Emergent = immediately. Urgent = within 48 hours. Nonurgent = later than 48 hours.

Figure 4-1 Red eye decision tree.
* = Potentially dangerous red eye: requires prompt, specialized care.

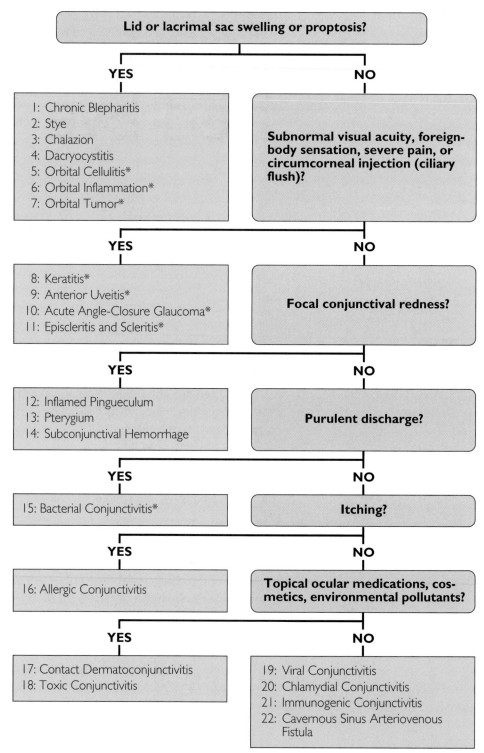

Lid or lacrimal sac swelling or proptosis?

YES

1: Chronic Blepharitis
2: Stye
3: Chalazion
4: Dacryocystitis
5: Orbital Cellulitis*
6: Orbital Inflammation*
7: Orbital Tumor*

NO

Subnormal visual acuity, foreign-body sensation, severe pain, or circumcorneal injection (ciliary flush)?

YES

8: Keratitis*
9: Anterior Uveitis*
10: Acute Angle-Closure Glaucoma*
11: Episcleritis and Scleritis*

NO

Focal conjunctival redness?

YES

12: Inflamed Pingueculum
13: Pterygium
14: Subconjunctival Hemorrhage

NO

Purulent discharge?

YES

15: Bacterial Conjunctivitis*

NO

Itching?

YES

16: Allergic Conjunctivitis

NO

Topical ocular medications, cosmetics, environmental pollutants?

YES

17: Contact Dermatoconjunctivitis
18: Toxic Conjunctivitis

NO

19: Viral Conjunctivitis
20: Chlamydial Conjunctivitis
21: Immunogenic Conjunctivitis
22: Cavernous Sinus Arteriovenous Fistula

Figure 4-2 Blepharitis. The lid margins are swollen, red, irregular, and laden with crusts. (Courtesy W.K. Kellogg Eye Center, University of Michigan.)

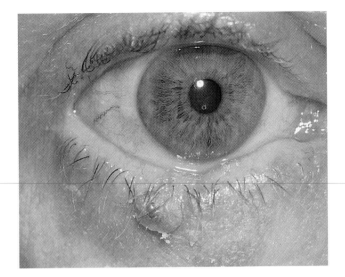

involving the conjunctiva or cornea (blepharokeratoconjunctivitis). Individuals who have rosacea or seborrheic dermatitis of the scalp and face are especially vulnerable to the posterior form of chronic blepharitis.

Clinical Presentation

☐ Gritty, burning sensation in eyes

☐ Mattering of eyes upon awakening

☐ Redness and swelling of lid margins

☐ Scaly, flaky debris on lid margins

☐ Mild conjunctival injection

☐ Face and scalp may show signs of rosacea or hyperkeratotic dermatitis

Treatment and Referral

☐ Instruct the patient to perform lid-margin scrubs twice a day as follows:
1. Place a warm washcloth over the closed lids for 5 minutes to soften the crusts.
2. Moisten a cotton-tipped applicator in a solution of 3 ounces of water and 3 drops of baby shampoo, and use it to scrub the closed lids.
3. Rinse the solution from the lids with clear water.
4. Brush off lid-margin debris with a clean, dry applicator.

☐ For anterior blepharitis, prescribe nightly application of bacitracin or erythromycin ointment.

- For posterior blepharitis, prescribe oral tetracycline 0.5 to 1 g/day in four doses or doxycycline 50 to 100 mg once or twice daily (except in pregnant patients and children aged 12 years or less).
- Continue this treatment until the symptoms and signs disappear.
- Refer nonurgently if the symptoms and signs do not respond after several weeks.

2: Stye

A stye, or external hordeolum, is an inflammation of the ciliary follicles or accessory glands of the anterior lid margin (Figure 4-3). Styes are common in a setting of chronic blepharitis. They may be confused with chalazion, orbital cellulitis, or dacryocystitis.

Clinical Presentation

- Painful, tender focal mounding of one eyelid developing over days, often with pustule formation
- Mild conjunctival injection

Treatment and Referral

- Instruct the patient to apply warm compresses to the affected eye twice daily.
- If chronic blepharitis is the underlying condition, treat as recommended for that condition.
- Refer if the mass fails to disappear after several months; surgical excision may be necessary.

Figure 4-3 Stye. The tender red mass near the lid margin was caused by inflamed lash follicles or sebaceous glands. Chalazion, caused by an inflamed meibomian gland, is similar but points toward the underlying conjunctiva.

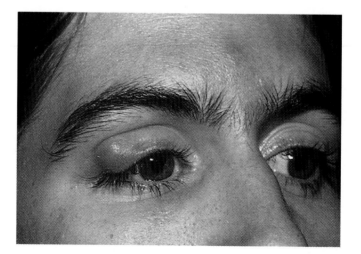

CLOSE-UP

FEATURES OF A DANGEROUS RED EYE

- ☐ Severe ocular pain
- ☐ Photophobia
- ☐ Persistent blurred vision
- ☐ Proptosis
- ☐ Reduced ocular movements
- ☐ Ciliary flush
- ☐ Irregular corneal light reflection

- ☐ Corneal epithelial defect or opacity
- ☐ Pupil unreactive to direct light
- ☐ Worsening signs after 3 days of pharmacologic treatment
- ☐ Compromised host: neonate, immunosuppressed patient, or soft contact lens wearer

3: Chalazion

A chalazion, or internal hordeolum, is an inflammation of the meibomian glands. It is deeper within lid tissue than a stye, but may be confused with stye, orbital cellulitis, or dacryocystitis.

Clinical Presentation

- ☐ Painful, focal tenderness of one eyelid developing over days; may not show external mounding, as the inflammation is deep within lid tissue
- ☐ Mild conjunctival injection

Treatment and Referral

- ☐ Instruct the patient to apply warm compresses to the affected eye twice daily.
- ☐ If chronic blepharitis is the underlying condition, treat as recommended above for posterior blepharitis.
- ☐ Refer if the mass fails to disappear after several months; surgical excision may be necessary. A persistent lid mass in an adult may be a sebaceous carcinoma.

4: Dacryocystitis

Dacryocystitis, or inflammation of the lacrimal sac, is generally caused by bacterial infection in the setting of an obstructed nasolacrimal passage (Figure 4-4). It is most common in infants whose nasolacrimal passage remains closed. In adults, the condition is the result of chronic sinusitis, facial trauma, or (rarely) neoplasm. (See "Tearing" in Chapter 3.) Its location in the medial lower lid usually allows the differentiation of dacryocystitis from stye, chalazion, or orbital cellulitis.

Figure 4-4 Dacryocystitis. The lacrimal sac is distended by infection.

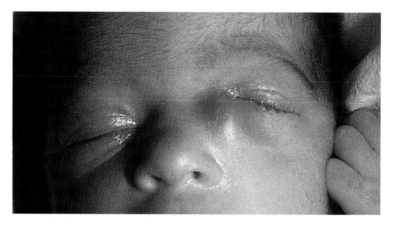

Clinical Presentation

- ☐ Mucopurulent discharge
- ☐ Excessive tearing
- ☐ Tender swelling of medial lower lid (overlying the lacrimal sac)
- ☐ Injection of surrounding palpebral conjunctiva and, to a lesser degree, bulbar conjunctiva
- ☐ Discharge from punctum sometimes elicited by pressing on lower lid mass

Treatment and Referral

- ☐ For infants, prescribe topical and oral antibiotics.
- ☐ Refer infants nonurgently if signs do not regress by 9 months of age; lacrimal probing may be necessary.
- ☐ Refer all adults nonurgently without treating; they may require surgery to open a passage for tears into the nose (dacryocystorhinostomy).

5: Orbital Cellulitis

Both forms of orbital cellulitis, preseptal and postseptal, are bacterial infections of periocular tissues (Figure 4-5). Preseptal cellulitis involves the soft tissues anterior to the orbital septum, a connective-tissue curtain that divides the anterior third from the posterior two thirds of the orbit. Postseptal cellulitis occurs posterior to this curtain of tissue.

Both kinds are rare in adults but common in children, originating in infected paranasal sinuses. In immunocompromised hosts, particularly diabetic patients, the physician must be alert to the possibility of mucormycosis or aspergillosis, life-threatening fungal infections that require prompt management.

Figure 4-5 Orbital cellulitis. The lids are swollen and violaceous, owing to orbital soft-tissue infection.

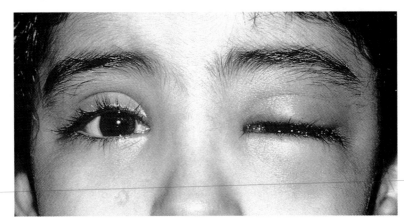

Preseptal infection may be confused with stye, chalazion, dacryocystitis, or infectious conjunctivitis. In normal adult hosts, signs of postseptal infection may mimic those of Graves' disease, orbital pseudotumor, and neoplasm.

Clinical Presentation

☐ Periocular pain

☐ Fever

☐ Symptoms of upper respiratory tract infection

☐ Violaceous swelling of upper and lower lids (usually unilateral)

☐ Mild, diffuse conjunctival injection

☐ Tenderness of lids and globe

☐ Reduced ocular movement (postseptal infection)

☐ Proptosis (postseptal infection)

☐ Visual loss (uncommon; only postseptal infection)

Treatment and Referral

☐ For children age 5 and younger, if signs suggest preseptal infection only, treat for presumed *Haemophilus influenzae* infection with intravenous antibiotics.

☐ For children over age 5 and adults, if signs suggest preseptal infection only, treat with oral antibiotics for skin and sinus bacterial organisms, *Staphylococcus aureus* and *Streptococcus pneumoniae*.

☐ For children and adults, if signs suggest postseptal infection, order sinoorbital imaging studies to rule out sinusitis, orbital subperiosteal abscess, or tumor.

□ For all ages, treat confirmed postseptal cellulitis with intravenous nafcillin and chloramphenicol or third-generation cephalosporins.

□ Lack of improvement in 24 to 48 hours signals either an incorrect diagnosis or ineffective antibacterial agents.

□ Consider fungal infections in immunocompromised hosts.

□ Consult an ophthalmologist and otorhinolaryngologist urgently for all cases. Orbital abscess may require surgical drainage.

6: Orbital Inflammation

Noninfectious, immunogenic conditions can inflame the orbital soft tissues, most commonly in Graves' disease (Figure 4-6) and idiopathic inflammation of the orbit (orbital pseudotumor). Conjunctival injection may be the only ophthalmic manifestation (see "Immunogenic Conjunctivitis" later in this chapter), but generally it is a surface sign of underlying inflammation of extraocular muscles, sclera, uvea, lacrimal gland, or orbital fat. Orbital manifestations often occur in patients who are chemically euthyroid.

Clinical Presentation

□ Pain

□ Proptosis

□ Tearing

□ Conjunctival injection

□ Mild mucoid discharge

□ Lid retraction, swelling, or ptosis

□ Diplopia

□ Visual loss

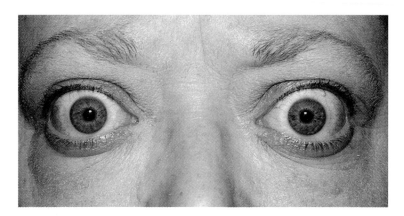

Figure 4-6 Graves' disease. The lids are retracted and the conjunctiva is hyperemic, reflecting inflammation of orbital soft tissues. (Courtesy W.K. Kellogg Eye Center, University of Michigan.)

CLOSE-UP

DANGERS OF CERTAIN DRUGS IN TREATING RED EYE

Do not use topical corticosteroids or corticosteroid-antibiotic combinations in treating a red eye. These agents may mask serious conditions and create others such as glaucoma, cataract, infection, and corneal perforation. The figure shows corneal perforation in a patient who had keratitis sicca and was treated long-term with topical corticosteroids.

Be prudent about prescribing topical decongestants, especially if the redness is not relieved promptly or if there are worrisome features.

See the Close-Up "Dangers of Anti-infectives + Cortico-steroids" in Chapter 7 for a warning on corticosteroid use.

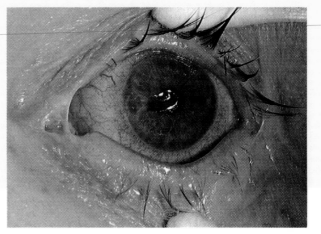

Courtesy W.K. Kellogg Eye Center, University of Michigan.

Treatment and Referral

☐ Order imaging studies to differentiate inflammation from tumor.

☐ Evaluate systemically if Graves' disease is likely. In Graves' disease, systemic corticosteroid treatment is generally reserved for optic neuropathy. Topical corticosteroid treatment is not recommended: it is ineffective and poses risks. (See the Close-Up "Dangers of Certain Drugs in Treating Red Eye.")

☐ Refer suspected orbital disease urgently.

7: Orbital Tumor

Tumors may involve the orbit primarily, by extension from paranasal sinuses, or secondarily, by metastasis. Diagnosis depends heavily on imaging.

Clinical Presentation

☐ Pain

☐ Proptosis (exophthalmos)

☐ Tearing

☐ Conjunctival injection or ecchymosis

- ☐ Ptosis
- ☐ Diplopia
- ☐ Visual loss

Treatment and Referral

- ☐ Order an imaging study (computed tomography or magnetic resonance imaging) to determine the location and extent of the tumor.
- ☐ Refer urgently for further management, which usually involves surgery unless the tumor is metastatic.

8: Keratitis

Keratitis (inflammation of the cornea) is most often caused by infection, trauma, dry eyes, ultraviolet exposure, contact lens overwear, or immunogenic states (Figure 4-7). Although far less common than conjunctivitis, keratitis must be recognized promptly because it may lead to permanent visual loss. (See also "Conjunctival and Corneal Foreign Bodies" in Chapter 5.) Some forms of keratitis begin with epithelial (surface) breakdown; infection may lead to corneal opacification, loss of tissue, perforation, and endophthalmitis. Many noninfectious forms of keratitis begin in deeper corneal layers, causing swelling and scarring. If the epithelium is not disrupted, fluorescein staining is normal.

Clinical Presentation

- ☐ Blurred vision
- ☐ Photophobia
- ☐ Periocular pain
- ☐ Foreign-body sensation (grittiness)
- ☐ Injection concentrated in circumcorneal, or limbal, region (ciliary flush)
- ☐ Fragmented corneal light reflection (sometimes)
- ☐ Corneal opacification (sometimes)

Treatment and Referral

- ☐ Do not attempt to treat. Refer emergently because of the complexity of diagnosis and the importance of specific treatment to prevent permanent loss of vision.

9: Anterior Uveitis

Anterior uveitis (iritis, iridocyclitis) represents inflammation of the iris and ciliary muscle (Figure 4-8). Like episcleritis and scleritis, anterior uveitis is an

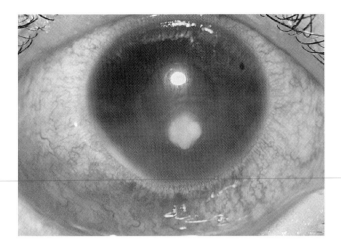

Figure 4-7 Bacterial keratitis. The white corneal opacity suggests purulence and necrosis. (Courtesy W.K. Kellogg Eye Center, University of Michigan.)

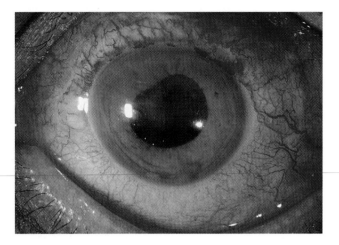

Figure 4-8 Anterior uveitis. The irregular pupil shape is caused by inflammatory adhesion of the iris margin to the anterior lens surface superiorly. (Courtesy W.K. Kellogg Eye Center, University of Michigan.)

autoimmune reaction that may be either isolated or part of a systemic state such as ankylosing spondylitis, juvenile rheumatoid arthritis, Reiter's syndrome, sarcoidosis, herpes simplex, herpes zoster, or Behcet's disease.

Clinical Presentation

☐ Periocular pain

☐ Photophobia

☐ Vision may be blurred but is often normal

☐ Circumcorneal conjunctival injection (ciliary flush)

☐ Irregular pupil, caused by adherence of the iris to the anterior lens or the posterior corneal surface

☐ Slit-lamp biomicroscopy reveals turbidity and cellular debris of the aqueous humor; cells may be adherent to the posterior surface of the cornea

☐ Intraocular pressure may be markedly elevated or depressed

Treatment and Referral

☐ Because the diagnosis depends on slit-lamp biomicroscopy, refer urgently for confirmation and treatment if clinical features are suggestive. Treatment by the ophthalmologist may include topical cycloplegics and corticosteroids, agents to lower intraocular pressure, and systemic corticosteroids in refractory cases.

Figure 4-9 Acute angle-closure glaucoma. Note the circumcorneal hyperemia (ciliary flush) and loss of corneal transparency. The sudden elevation of intraocular pressure causes failure of the metabolic pump that prevents aqueous humor from entering the cornea.

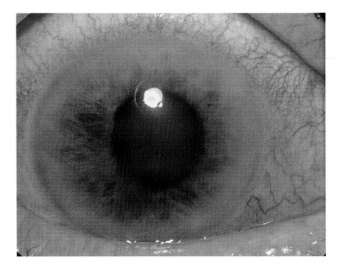

10: Acute Angle-Closure Glaucoma

Acute angle-closure glaucoma is an ophthalmic emergency associated with a sudden elevation in intraocular pressure (Figure 4-9). Arising from a blockage in the outflow of aqueous humor, it is a rare condition, most often occurring in middle-aged or older patients with anatomically small anterior chambers or altered iris structure. (Refer to "Acute Persistent Visual Loss" in Chapter 3 and Table 3-1 for additional diagnostic information. See also "Glaucoma" in Chapter 9.)

The vast majority of angle-closure incidents occur spontaneously. Very few cases are precipitated by topical pupil-dilating parasympatholytics, and virtually none by orally administered parasympatholytics—despite the drug-insert warnings.

Clinical Presentation

☐   Acute periocular pain; may be very severe and associated with nausea and vomiting, misdirecting attention to an abdominal source

☐   Acute photophobia

☐   Blurred vision

☐   Circumcorneal injection (ciliary flush)

☐   Corneal clouding

☐   Pupil unreactive to direct light

☐   Markedly elevated intraocular pressure (see the Close-Up "Diagnosis of Acute Angle-Closure Glaucoma")

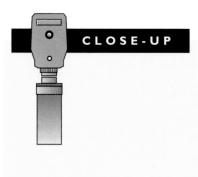

DIAGNOSIS OF ACUTE ANGLE-CLOSURE GLAUCOMA

The diagnosis of acute angle-closure glaucoma depends on finding elevated intraocular pressure. Applanation tonometry is much more accurate in this task than is indentation (Schiotz) tonometry or digital palpation of the globe. Physicians who do not habitually perform applanation tonometry should therefore pay particular attention to other typical findings and, if present, make a presumptive diagnosis, treat, and refer emergently.

Treatment and Referral

- ☐ If clinical features are suggestive, attempt to lower intraocular pressure quickly by instilling topical pilocarpine 2% every 5 minutes for three doses and topical timolol 0.5% one dose, and administering acetazolamide 500 mg one dose by mouth or vein.

- ☐ Refer emergently for further diagnosis and treatment. Once pressure is lowered, laser or surgical iridectomy may be performed by an ophthalmologist.

II: Episcleritis and Scleritis

Episcleritis is a focal inflammation of the deep subconjunctival (episcleral) tissue (Figure 4-10). Scleritis is a focal or diffuse inflammation of the sclera. Both conditions may have an autoimmune basis, but their associations with systemic states differ somewhat. Scleritis is nearly always associated with a necrotizing systemic vasculitis, often rheumatoid arthritis. Episcleritis is frequently an isolated condition, but may be seen in a variety of viral and idiopathic autoimmune conditions. While episcleritis has no severe ocular consequences, scleritis may cause extreme thinning ("melting") of the cornea or sclera and even perforation of the globe. Either condition may be confused with inflamed pingueculum, pterygium, foreign body, or tumor.

Clinical Presentation

- ☐ Eye pain, especially severe with scleritis
- ☐ Focal or, less commonly, diffuse bulbar conjunctival and episcleral injection
- ☐ In scleritis, scleral thinning may be extreme enough to allow the dark purple color of the underlying uvea to show through
- ☐ May be accompanied by keratitis and uveitis
- ☐ May be associated with a systemic autoimmune or viral condition

Figure 4-10 Episcleritis. Focal erythematous swelling of the bulbar conjunctiva and episcleral tissue.

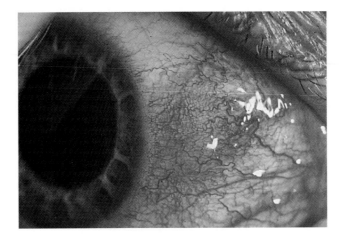

Treatment and Referral

☐ Refer urgently if either episcleritis or scleritis is suspected; the distinction between these conditions may be difficult to determine, even with slit-lamp biomicroscopy, and treatment may present problems as well. The ophthalmologist often first prescribes topical corticosteroids for scleritis, but may need to employ systemic corticosteroids or cytotoxic agents. Threatened ocular perforation in scleritis may require surgical patch grafts.

12: Inflamed Pingueculum

A pingueculum is an area of nasal or temporal bulbar conjunctiva that contains epithelial hyperplasia, probably in response to irritation from excessive sun and wind exposure (Figure 4-11). For unexplained reasons, it occasionally becomes inflamed for periods of weeks. Diagnostically, an inflamed pingueculum may be confused with episcleritis, scleritis, conjunctival tumor, or pterygium.

Clinical Presentation

☐ Mild ocular discomfort

☐ Focal conjunctival injection over a mounded area in the nasal or temporal canthus

Treatment and Referral

☐ Prescribe topical vasoconstrictors (see the Close-Up "Dangers of Certain Drugs in Treating Red Eye").

☐ Refer nonurgently if unresponsive after 1 week.

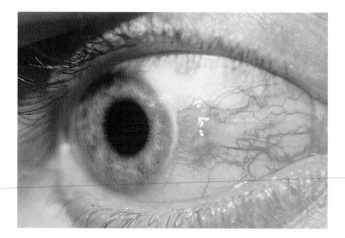

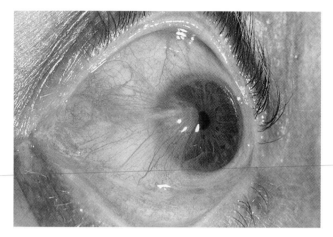

Figure 4-11 Inflamed pingueculum. Focal erythematous swelling of the bulbar conjunctiva. Resembles episcleritis, but is more discrete.

Figure 4-12 Pterygium. Hyperplasia and migration of conjunctiva onto the corneal surface.

13: Pterygium

A pterygium ("winged growth") is a fibrovascular proliferation of the nasal or, rarely, temporal bulbar conjunctiva (Figure 4-12). It grows toward the cornea and over its surface. If pain is a symptom, pterygium may be confused with inflamed pingueculum.

Clinical Presentation

☐ Usually painless

☐ Blurred vision (sometimes)

☐ Mounded, injected conjunctival tissue emanating from either canthus and abutting or invading the cornea

Treatment and Referral

☐ No medical treatment is satisfactory.

☐ Refer nonurgently unless the growth is long-standing, unchanging, and not causing any symptoms. If the pterygium is growing onto the cornea, it may have to be surgically excised.

14: Subconjunctival Hemorrhage

Subconjunctival hemorrhage not caused by direct ocular trauma is usually the result of a sudden increase in intrathoracic pressure, as in sneezing, coughing, or straining to evacuate (Figure 4-13). The weak-walled conjunctival vessels are liable to burst, especially in the elderly. Other causes are systemic hypertension and blood dyscrasias. Usually, no cause is identified. In neonates, subconjunctival hemorrhage is a common and benign consequence of vaginal delivery.

Clinical Presentation

☐   Blotchy (extravascular) bulbar conjunctival redness

Treatment and Referral

☐   No treatment is necessary.

☐   Measure blood pressure and investigate for blood dyscrasia if the hemorrhage is recurrent or the patient has no history of Valsalva's maneuver.

☐   Refer under the following circumstances:
   1.   The diagnosis is in doubt.
   2.   Some other abnormality becomes evident on the ophthalmic screening examination.

15: Bacterial Conjunctivitis

Bacterial conjunctivitis is a relatively unusual cause of red eye in normal hosts (Figure 4-14). The condition is generally self-limited, causes no permanent damage, and is not nearly as contagious as viral conjunctivitis. However, bacterial conjunctivitis in newborns must be diagnosed and treated promptly to prevent blindness. (See Table 4-1 and the Close-Up "Red Eye in Infants.")

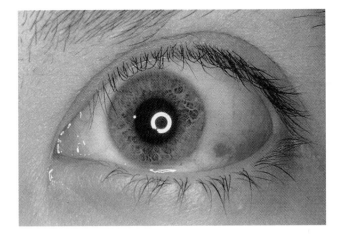

Figure 4-13 Subconjunctival hemorrhage. A conjunctival vessel has burst, due to Valsalva's maneuver, trauma, systemic hypertension, or blood dyscrasia.

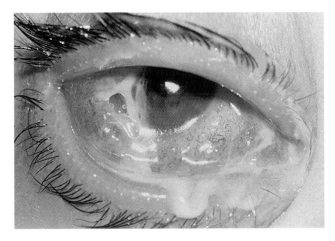

Figure 4-14 Bacterial conjunctivitis. The purulent discharge is distinctive.

TABLE 4-1
Treatment of Red Eye in Infants

Cause	Characteristics	Treatment
Chlamydia	About 80% of infectious red eyes in infants Onset day 2 to week 8 Mild to severe Organisms seen on direct fluorescent antibody stain of conjunctival scrapings Associated pneumonia common Rarely causes ocular damage even untreated	Tetracycline ointment qid for 4 weeks; oral erythromycin for 4 weeks Treat parents with oral doxycycline or erythromycin for 4 weeks
Neisseria gonorrhoeae	Less than 5% of infectious red eyes in infants Onset day 2 to 4 Usually hyperacute, but may be mild initially Purulent discharge Gram-negative intracellular cocci on scrapings; cultures confirm Inadequate treatment leads to corneal perforation and blindness	Topical aqueous penicillin 20,000 units/ml, 1 drop hourly; intravenous aqueous penicillin 50,000 units daily or ceftriaxone 50 to 75 mg/kg/day for 7 days
Staphylococcus, Streptococcus, gram-negative bacteria	Uncommon Onset usually after 5 days, but may be earlier Mucopurulent discharge May be associated with sepsis Can lead to corneal perforation Diagnosis by smear and culture	G+ organisms and *Haemophilus*: erythromycin ointment 6 times daily Other G− organisms: topical gentamicin every 1 to 2 hours
Herpes simplex	Uncommon Onset day 5 to 10 Usually type 2 Watery discharge Lid often swollen May be associated with mucocutaneous vesicles, systemic (including choroid, central nervous system) involvement Conjunctival smears show absence of polymorphonuclear leukocytes Viral cultures definitive	Topical trifluridine, vidarabine, or idoxuridine qh Intravenous acyclovir
Silver nitrate	Common but mild Resolves within 24 hours	None

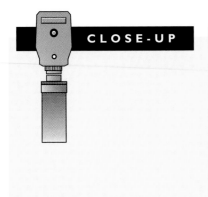

RED EYE IN INFANTS

Red eye in infants (*ophthalmia neonatorum*) is caused either by a mild, transitory chemical irritation owing to silver-nitrate prophylaxis or by an infectious process acquired in the birth canal. Affecting about 6% of infants, the infectious process is caused by *Chlamydia, Neisseria gonorrhoeae,* other bacteria, or herpes simplex. It is a challenging management problem because (1) the clinical signs are not distinctive; (2) the conjunctivitis may be a manifestation of systemic infection; and (3) untreated conjunctivitis may lead to blindness. Table 4-1 presents causes, characteristics, and treatment of red eye in infants.

Clinical Presentation

☐ Diffuse and marked conjunctival injection

☐ Purulent discharge

☐ Preauricular nodes usually not swollen

☐ Most common pathogens: *Staphylococcus aureus, Streptococcus pneumoniae,* and *Haemophilus influenzae*

Treatment and Referral

☐ Perform conjunctival scraping for smears and cultures in all affected infants and in immunocompromised hosts.

☐ For mild bacterial conjunctivitis, prescribe topical sulfa (acceptable as the least expensive first-line medication in nonallergic individuals).

☐ As an alternative to sulfa, prescribe an aminoglycoside (gentamicin, tobramycin), quinolone (ciprofloxacin, norfloxacin), or a combination antibiotic (neomycin–bacitracin–polymyxin B, trimethoprim–polymyxin B).

☐ For *Neisseria gonorrhoeae* conjunctivitis, prescribe topical aqueous penicillin (20,000 units/ml, 1 drop hourly) and intravenous penicillin (50,000 units daily) or intravenous ceftriaxone 50 to 75 mg/kg/day for 7 days. This treatment is emergent in newborns.

☐ Once the diagnosis of bacterial conjunctivitis has been made, quarantine is not necessary because of the low degree of contagion.

☐ Refer emergently under the following circumstances:
   1. *Neisseria* conjunctivitis is suspected.
   2. The patient uses extended-wear (overnight) contact lenses (the concern is keratitis, particularly that caused by *Pseudomonas aeruginosa* or *Acanthamoeba*).
   3. There has been recent eye surgery.

□ Refer urgently under the following circumstances:
  1. The signs worsen after 3 days of treatment or there is no improvement after 7 days.
  2. The host is immunocompromised.
  3. There is a history of injury with a foreign body (the concern is an unusual pathogen conveyed with a foreign body).

16: Allergic Conjunctivitis

Allergic conjunctivitis is part of a systemic atopic reaction of all mucous membranes to a systemic allergen, usually airborne (Figure 4-15). Therefore, it is usually seasonal and tends to follow the course of upper respiratory tract symptoms. Sometimes, however, it may be the leading—or only—allergic manifestation.

Clinical Presentation

□ Diffuse conjunctival injection

□ Prominent itching (pruritus)

□ Boggy (edematous) conjunctiva

□ Stringy, mucoid discharge

□ Always bilateral

Treatment and Referral

□ Prescribe topical decongestants (see the Close-Up "Dangers of Certain Drugs in Treating Red Eye" in this chapter, and Chapter 7).

□ Prescribe systemic antihistamines.

□ Treat the systemic allergy (desensitization, removal of allergens).

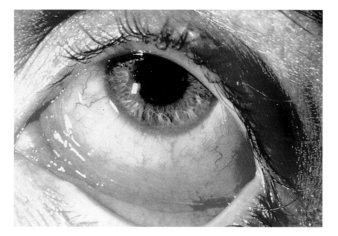

Figure 4-15 Allergic conjunctivitis. A boggy, hyperemic conjunctiva accompanied by lid swelling and itching is distinctive.

□ Refer nonurgently only if the symptoms and signs are unresponsive to the treatment regimen.

17: Contact Dermatoconjunctivitis

Contact dermatoconjunctivitis is caused by an allergic reaction to topically applied medications (Figure 4-16). By far the most common offender is neomycin (10% of patients treated with this agent).

Clinical Presentation

□ History of instillation of eyedrops or ointment (especially aminoglycosides, atropine)

□ History of disappearance of symptoms when the offending medication is discontinued

□ Diffuse conjunctival injection

□ Erythema, swelling of eyelids

Treatment and Referral

□ Discontinue the offending medication.

□ Refer nonurgently if the symptoms and signs fail to respond after 1 week.

18: Toxic Conjunctivitis

Toxic conjunctivitis is usually caused by topical ocular medications or cosmetics. Nearly every medication has been implicated, including aerosolized chemicals, although usually only after exposure to a high dose. The physician must beware of making this diagnosis if the real cause is chronic infectious conjunctivitis, uveitis, scleritis, or blepharitis.

Figure 4-16 Contact dermatoconjunctivitis. Eczematous changes in the lids accompany this red eye.

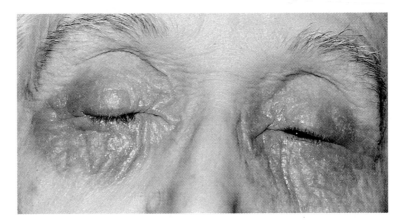

Clinical Presentation

- History of use of topical ocular medications or cosmetics or of exposure to environmental pollutants
- Mild but persistent ocular discomfort
- Sticky eyelids upon awakening
- Diffuse conjunctival injection, but barely visible

Treatment and Referral

- Eliminate the offending agent, which may be difficult to identify unless it is applied directly to the conjunctiva or eyelids.
- Prescribe topical vasoconstrictors, if necessary (see the Close-Up "Dangers of Certain Drugs in Treating Red Eye").
- Refer nonurgently if the conjunctival injection fails to respond after 1 week.

19: Viral Conjunctivitis

Viral conjunctivitis is the most common cause of an acute red eye (Figure 4-17). Fortunately, viral conjunctivitis is usually a self-limited infection that leaves no permanent damage. Caused most often by adenovirus species, it cannot be treated effectively with antimicrobial agents. Instead, management is directed at scrupulous hygiene to prevent the spread of these highly contagious organisms. Contagion is most likely when discharge is present.

Clinical Presentation

- Isolated or part of systemic viral syndrome
- Often a history of exposure to an infected person (incubation period is about 8 days)

Figure 4-17 Viral conjunctivitis. A watery discharge and diffuse injection are characteristic.

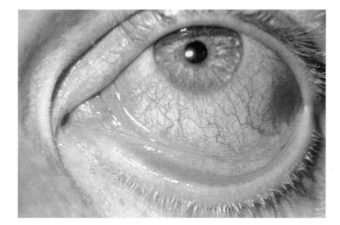

- Ocular discomfort, rather than pain
- Diffuse conjunctival injection
- Watery discharge
- Tender preauricular node
- Monocular or binocular involvement
- Keratitis in some patients, producing slightly degraded vision, foreign-body sensation, and photophobia

Treatment and Referral

- Do not prescribe anti-infectives: they are ineffective, and their application may lead to further contamination and viral spread.
- Instruct patients to wash their hands frequently and avoid touching their eyes and sharing towels.
- Advise patients to avoid communal activities (eg, work, school, daycare) as long as discharge is present.
- Refer urgently under the following circumstances:
  1. The diagnosis is in question.
  2. Symptoms appear to worsen.
  3. Keratitis is suspected or diagnosed.

20: Chlamydial Conjunctivitis

Chlamydial conjunctivitis occurs in two forms: (1) neonatal, acquired from an infected cervix; and (2) adult, acquired by sexual contact (Figure 4-18). The neonatal form, the most common cause of red eye in a newborn, often cannot be clinically distinguished from other causes. (See the Close-Up "Red Eye in Infants" and Table 4-1.) The adult form consists of a chronic, usually indolent conjunctivitis that is resistant to standard topical antibiotics.

Clinical Presentation

- Injected conjunctiva with follicles
- Mucopurulent discharge
- In infants, onset from day 2 to week 8 after birth
- May be monocular or binocular
- Signs vary from mild to severe and are not distinctive
- Diagnostic finding of typical elementary bodies on direct fluorescent antibody stain of conjunctival scrapings; culture also possible but result delayed
- Associated pneumonia common in infants

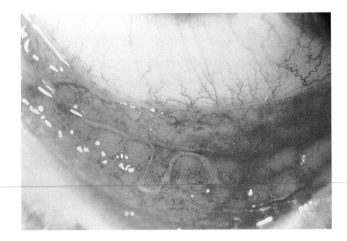

Figure 4-18 Chlamydial conjunctivitis. The inferior bulbar and palpebral conjunctiva is commonly affected with a chronic, follicular inflammation.

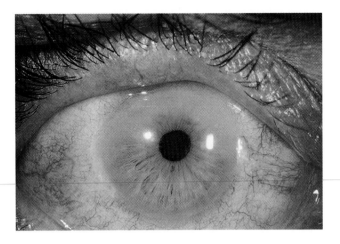

Figure 4-19 Immunogenic conjunctivitis (Wegener's granulomatosis). A low-grade conjunctival infection is accompanied by marginal keratitis and eyelid swelling. (Courtesy W.K. Kellogg Eye Center, University of Michigan.)

Treatment and Referral

☐ Send conjunctival scraping in *Chlamydia* collection kit to microbiology laboratory to search for elementary bodies found on direct fluorescent antibody stain.

☐ For neonates, prescribe topical tetracycline ointment 4 times daily for 4 weeks and oral erythromycin for 4 weeks.

☐ For adults, prescribe oral doxycycline or erythromycin for 4 weeks.

☐ Treat parents and sexual partners with adult regimen.

☐ Refer infants urgently and adults nonurgently if conjunctivitis does not improve or worsens after 5 days of treatment.

☐ Refer adults nonurgently if conjunctivitis lingers after treatment ends.

21: Immunogenic Conjunctivitis

Immunogenic conjunctivitis is a noninfectious inflammation found in association with systemic disorders of the immune system, such as Graves' disease, rheumatoid arthritis, Sjogren's syndrome, lupus erythematosus, Wegener's granulomatosis, relapsing polychondritis, and polyarteritis nodosa (Figure 4-19).

Clinical Presentation

☐ May have no ocular symptoms unless orbitopathy, keratitis, uveitis, or scleritis coexists

□ Minimal mucoid conjunctival discharge

□ Chronic, low-grade, diffuse conjunctival injection

□ Systemic immunogenic condition has usually been recognized, but conjunctivitis may be an early and isolated manifestation

Treatment and Referral

□ Aim treatment at the underlying condition.

□ Refer nonurgently for ophthalmologic evaluation to exclude other causes.

22: Cavernous Sinus Arteriovenous Fistula

Conjunctival hyperemia (without inflammation) may result from the increased orbital venous pressure owing to an arteriovenous (AV) shunt (fistula) in the cavernous sinus (Figure 4-20). Cavernous sinus AV fistulas may be caused by head trauma or may occur spontaneously, especially in postmenopausal women. Low-flow (dural) fistulas may close without treatment; high-flow fistulas may require endovascular procedures.

Clinical Presentation

□ Chronic, diffuse conjunctival hyperemia, usually monocular

□ Achy periocular pain rather than the discomfort that is typical of infectious conjunctivitis

□ May have proptosis, ptosis, elevated intraocular pressure, diplopia, visual loss

□ Some patients hear a "whooshing" sound synchronous with their pulse

Treatment and Referral

□ Refer nonurgently to an ophthalmologist for confirmation of the diagnosis. Management may involve endovascular embolization done by a radiologist.

Figure 4-20 Arteriovenous fistula (cavernous sinus). Corkscrew dilation of conjunctival vessels is distinctive. (Courtesy W.K. Kellogg Eye Center, University of Michigan.)

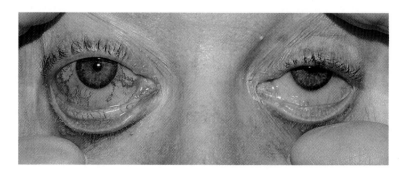

CHAPTER 5

Ophthalmic Trauma

The physician plays an important role in the management of four ophthalmic trauma problems: chemical burn; blunt or lacerating injury; intraocular foreign body; and conjunctival or corneal foreign body. This chapter presents the basic information that enables the physician to care for patients presenting with these eye injuries. Because so much ophthalmic trauma requires quick and decisive action, the Close-Up "Management of Ophthalmic Trauma" is provided as a ready reference.

Chemical Burn

Chemical burns to the eye are vision-threatening emergencies that require immediate, on-site treatment. Among the most dangerous burns are those from alkali-containing products such as household cleaners, fertilizers, and pesticides (Figure 5-1). If not treated promptly, alkali burns can cause irreversible damage to the cornea and permanent loss of vision. Burns from acidic agents, such as car battery fluid, are also potentially harmful and warrant immediate attention. Other chemicals cause milder, reversible damage.

History-Taking

☐ **Do not spend time taking a detailed history.**
As soon as you know that a chemical has contacted the eye, institute emergency management.

CLOSE-UP

PATCHES AND SHIELDS

Pressure-patch the eye for comfort; shield the eye for protection.

Patching is indicated for a noninfected corneal abrasion to prevent blinking, during which the inner surface of the lid irritates the exposed trigeminal nerve endings. If the cornea may be infected, the eye is not patched because blinking promotes natural cleansing. For most abrasions, 1 day's wear is sufficient. Most effective is a double patch, consisting of an internal, folded, oval patch and an external, unfolded patch.

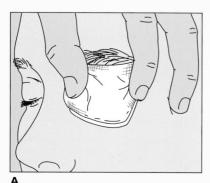

A

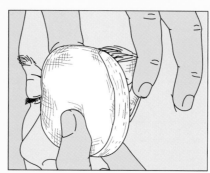

B

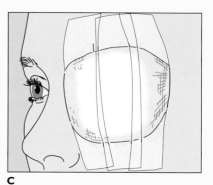

C

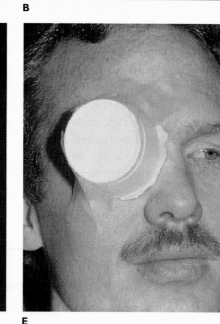

D

E

1. Fold an eye patch and apply it to the closed lid (Figure A).

2. Apply an unfolded eye patch over the folded patch (Figure B).

3. Tape the patch firmly to the forehead and zygoma (Figure C). The tape should not extend to the mandible because jaw movement could loosen the patch.

Shield any contusion or laceration of the globe or its adnexal structures to protect these tissues from further contact. Always shield a suspected ruptured globe. A fenestrated aluminum (Fox) shield is best (Figure D), but a homemade shield may be fashioned by trimming a paper cup (Figure E).

7. If you find corneal epithelial defects, instill a topical antibiotic (such as sulfacetamide or gentamicin) and a cycloplegic (such as cyclopentolate 1%), and pressure-patch the eye (see the Close-Up "Patches and Shields").

Referral

☐ Refer immediately after treatment if you find one or more of the following:
   1. Acid or alkali burn
   2. Subnormal visual acuity
   3. Severe conjunctival swelling
   4. Corneal clouding

☐ Refer all other patients within 24 hours.

Blunt or Lacerating Injury

Laceration of the ocular adnexa or globe is one of the most serious injuries. Blunt trauma, associated with fights, automobile accidents, and sports accidents, also may result in serious damage (Figure 5-3). Most often, blunt trauma causes contusion, but with strong impact the tissues may be torn.

A ruptured globe is the most dangerous consequence of either blunt trauma or laceration. Intraocular hemorrhage and retinal detachment also may have serious visual consequences. Less dangerous—but still potentially serious—are complicated lacerations of the eyelids. Contusions limited to the orbital tissues and fractures of the orbital walls are much less threatening to vision, but they may involve serious coincident facial and intracranial injuries. Because lacerations of the globe may be difficult to find (Figure 5-4), the physician should presume a ruptured globe if a history or evidence of severe trauma exists.

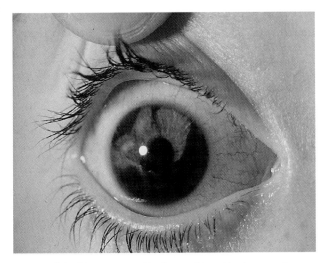

Figure 5-3 Blunt trauma. Hyphema (blood in the anterior chamber) and an iris defect are evidence of severe injury. (Courtesy W.K. Kellogg Eye Center, University of Michigan.)

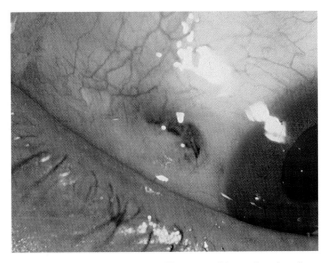

Figure 5-4 Lacerating trauma. The wound is small and easily overlooked.

History-Taking

- **What object struck or was used to strike the patient?**
  Differentiates sharp from blunt trauma.

- **Where did the blow strike the patient (eye, forehead, cheek)?**
  If the eye took the blow, visual consequences are likely to be greater.

- **How hard was the blow (pain, "saw stars," fell to ground, lost consciousness)?**
  Helps to determine the likelihood of serious ocular or periocular injury.

- **How long ago did the blow occur?**
  The longer a globe has been ruptured, the greater the likelihood of intraocular infection.

- **Does the patient complain of decreased visual acuity or visual field, diplopia, or severe pain?**
  Indirectly assesses seriousness of ocular or periocular injury.

Examination and Treatment

1. Test visual acuity by the Snellen method or with a near vision card. Do not test if doing so would require forcing the lids open or instilling anesthetic.

2. Inspect for lid lacerations and proptosis (suggesting retrobulbar hemorrhage). Check for the four characteristics of complicated lid lacerations that warrant immediate referral to an ophthalmologist:
   a. Deep lacerations possibly involving the globe
   b. Large lacerations with fat prolapse or with tissue loss requiring complicated repair techniques
   c. Lacerations extending to the lid margins that can lead to physical deformities if not repaired properly (Figure 5-5)
   d. Lacerations involving the nasolacrimal system that can lead to permanent tearing if not repaired properly

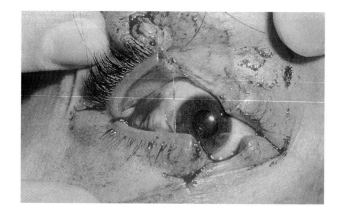

Figure 5-5 Complicated lid laceration. The upper and lower lids have defects extending to the margins. Imperfect repair will result in functional and cosmetic deformities.

MANAGEMENT OF HYPHEMA

Hyphema, or blood in the anterior chamber of the eye, is most often caused by trauma to the vessels at the root of the iris. The figure shows blood filling the lower part of the anterior chamber. Hyphema is an important sign for two reasons: (1) the globe may have sustained other, even more vision-threatening contusion injury; and (2) rebleeding can occur in up to 30% of cases, possibly leading to blinding elevation of intraocular pressure and the need for emergency surgical evacuation of the clot.

The finding of hyphema requires an eye shield and immediate referral to an ophthalmologist. The management of hyphema is aimed at ruling out treatable concomitant injuries and preventing rebleeding. Although antifibrinolytics (aminocaproic acid, tranexamic acid) are considered effective in reducing the chances of rebleeding, most ophthalmologists simply recommend a shield, reduction in physical activities, and frequent re-examination within the first 5 days. To accomplish these goals, hospitalization, especially of children, is sometimes necessary.

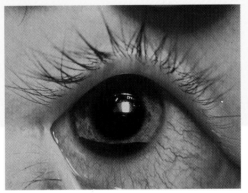

Courtesy W.K. Kellogg Eye Center, University of Michigan.

3. Check ocular movements and alignment (corneal reflections, cover test). Misalignment or decreased eye movement suggests an orbital wall fracture.

4. If the lids do not obscure the globe, inspect for severe conjunctival ecchymosis and swelling, corneal or scleral laceration, irregular pupil, deformed globe, or hyphema (see the Close-Up "Management of Hyphema"). **Caution:** Do not forcibly retract the lids and possibly put pressure on a ruptured globe, causing extrusion of its contents.

5. If you find or suspect any of the above conditions, shield the eye and refer immediately (see the Close-Up "Patches and Shields"). The shield protects the eye and surrounding tissues from further manipulation and injury. **Caution:** Do not patch the eye, as a patch might exert unwanted pressure.

6. In the absence of severe contusion or lacerations of the globe, repair uncomplicated lid lacerations as follows:
    a. Cleanse the wound with a standard antiseptic solution.
    b. Close the skin with interrupted 6-0 silk or polyglactin (Vicryl) sutures.

Referral

☐ Shield the globe and refer immediately after inspection if you find one or more of the following:

1. Severe pain
2. Subnormal visual acuity
3. Severe conjunctival ecchymosis
4. Hyphema
5. Irregular pupil
6. Corneal or scleral laceration
7. Deformed globe
8. Complicated lid laceration

☐ Shield the globe and refer within 24 hours if none of the above findings is present but reduced ocular movements suggest contusion of the globe or an orbital wall fracture.

☐ Refer within 48 hours if you suspect mild contusion limited to the orbital soft tissues.

Intraocular Foreign Body

High-velocity missiles, such as metal bits released by drilling or hammering and shotgun or BB pellets, can penetrate the globe without causing severe pain, obvious physical signs, or early visual disturbances (Figure 5-6). Nevertheless,

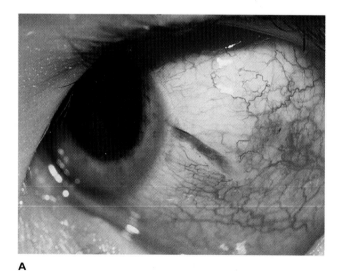
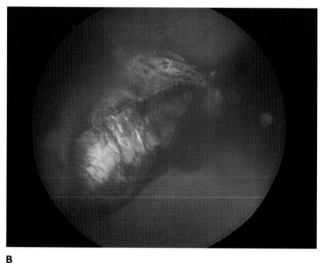

A   **B**

Figure 5-6 Intraocular foreign body. (**A**) The entrance wound. (**B**) A foreign body in the vitreous, seen through the pupil. (Courtesy W.K. Kellogg Eye Center, University of Michigan.)

prompt evaluation and removal, if possible, of an intraocular foreign body are critical. If undetected or allowed to remain in place, such objects can induce serious sequelae that threaten vision and impede their removal. For example, a penetrated lens will rapidly develop a cataract, and torn retinal vessels will gradually bleed into the vitreous cavity. Because physical signs may be slight, the physician must rely on history-taking to make a presumptive diagnosis.

History-Taking

- **Was the patient doing metal-on-metal hammering, drilling, or sawing?**
  The most common settings for an intraocular foreign body.

- **Was the patient exposed to a high-speed missile?**
  Heightens the suspicion of an intraocular foreign body.

- **Did the patient feel a sudden impact on the eyelids or eye?**
  Suggests contact, if not penetration.

- **Does the patient complain of pain or decreased vision?**
  Increases the likelihood of intraocular penetration.

- **Was the patient wearing glasses or goggles?**
  Reduces the risk of intraocular penetration.

Examination and Treatment

1. Test visual acuity by the Snellen method or with the near vision card. Do not test if doing so would require forcing the lids apart.

2. Inspect for small lacerations or holes in the eyelids.

3. Inspect for corneal or scleral laceration, hyphema, irregular pupil, or absent red reflex (see the Close-Up "Management of Ophthalmic Trauma").

Referral

- Refer immediately if the history suggests strongly that the eye was struck by a high-speed missile, even if there are no physical signs.

Conjunctival and Corneal Foreign Bodies

Conjunctival and corneal foreign bodies are usually airborne debris that blow into the eye (Figure 5-7). The patient will report that "there is something in my eye" and that the eye is tearing and light-sensitive. Although foreign bodies are sometimes difficult to remove, with proper technique the physician often can find and remove some corneal foreign bodies and conjunctival foreign bodies that lodge in the tarsal sulcus under the upper eyelid. If the foreign body has injured the cornea, patients will also require followup care for corneal abrasion.

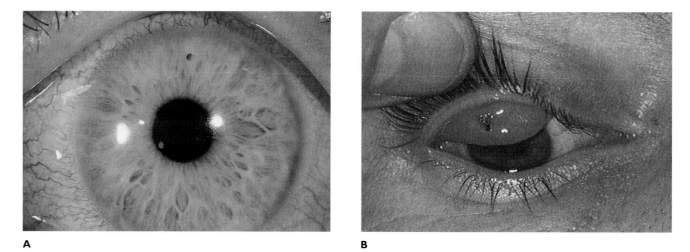

Figure 5-7 Foreign bodies. (**A**) A corneal foreign body. (**B**) A tarsal (conjunctival) foreign body. (Part A courtesy W.K. Kellogg Eye Center, University of Michigan.)

If the patient did not develop the foreign-body sensation acutely, but noted its onset upon awakening or gradually during the day, suspect an infectious keratitis (herpes simplex or other microorganisms). In a contact lens wearer, the condition may be either keratitis due to overwear or a serious infection with *Pseudomonas aeruginosa*. If the patient was struck by a high-speed missile, the foreign body may have entered the globe. This situation requires entirely different management (see "Intraocular Foreign Body" above).

History-Taking

☐ **Does the patient think that a particle "blew into" the eye, or could the patient have been struck by a high-speed missile?**
Helps to differentiate surface from intraocular foreign body.

☐ **Did the foreign-body sensation begin slowly or upon awakening, rather than suddenly?**
Helps to differentiate infectious keratitis from surface foreign body.

Examination and Treatment

1. Test visual acuity by the Snellen method or with the near vision card. If necessary, instill a topical anesthetic to induce comfort and cooperation.
2. Under magnification and bright light, inspect the corneal and conjunctival surfaces for a foreign body. To inspect the conjunctiva of the upper lid, evert the lid as follows:
   a. Instruct the patient to look down.
   b. With the fingers of your nondominant hand, grasp the eyelashes of the upper lid and pull the lid down and away from the eye (Figure 5-8A).

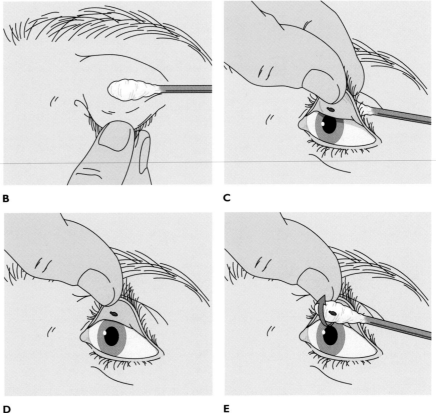

A B C

D E

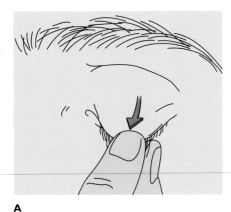

Figure 5-8 Eversion of the upper lid and removal of a tarsal foreign body. (**A**) After instructing the patient to look down, grasp the eyelashes of the upper lid and pull down and away from the eye. (**B**) With the other hand, place a moistened applicator in the upper lid fold, 1/2 inch above the lid margin. (**C**) Evert the upper lid over the applicator. (**D**) Remove the applicator, keeping the upper lid everted with your thumb. (**E**) Inspect the tarsal conjunctiva with a penlight and remove the foreign body by using a rolling motion of the applicator.

    c. With the dominant hand, place a moistened cotton-tipped applicator horizontally across the skin crease of the eyelid, approximately ½ inch above the lid margin (Figure 5-8B).

    d. With the opposite hand, fold (evert) the upper lid over the applicator to expose the underlying conjunctival surface (Figure 5-8C).

    e. Draw the applicator stick out toward the temple, but keep the upper lid in the everted position using the thumb of the opposite hand (Figure 5-8D).

3. Remove the foreign body by rolling the moistened cotton-tipped applicator across the corneal or conjunctival surface (Figure 5-8E). If this maneuver is unsuccessful, a corneal foreign body can sometimes be nudged out under adequate light and magnification with the side of a 22- or 25-gauge needle. (This procedure should be done only by someone with experience.) Rust rings need not be removed; they generally disappear in the healing phase.

4. After removing the foreign body, stain the cornea with fluorescein and inspect it under cobalt-blue light or a Wood's lamp for green spots or lines, which signify corneal epithelial defects.

5. If you find corneal epithelial defects, instill a topical antibiotic (such as sulfacetamide or gentamicin) and a cycloplegic (such as cyclopentolate 1%), and pressure-patch the eye (see the Close-Up "Patches and Shields").

6. Schedule a visit within 24 hours to confirm epithelial healing without infection, or refer to an ophthalmologist for followup.

Referral

□ Shield the eye and refer immediately any patient with a corneal or conjunctival foreign body that cannot be dislodged with a moistened cotton-tipped applicator or the side of a needle.

□ Refer within 24 hours any patient with a large corneal abrasion or a foreign-body sensation if no foreign body is detected.

CLOSE-UP

PREVENTION OF EYE INJURIES

Countless preventable eye injuries occur every year. The physician can play a major role in preventing ophthalmic trauma by instructing patients—particularly those with only one functional eye—to take the following precautions:

□ Wear protective eye guards or spectacles (see the figure) when playing rough contact sports (hockey, football, basketball), engaging in sports that involve missiles (baseball, lacrosse) or racquets (tennis, racquetball, squash), and pursuing occupations (carpentry, metal work) in which eye trauma is likely. Protective goggles should carry a label certifying that they meet the safety specifications of the American National Standards Institute (ANSI). Spectacles made of polycarbonate plastic lenses with a minimum center thickness of 3 mm and industrial-strength frames are considered most protective.

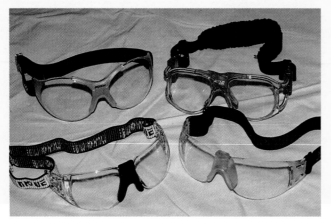

□ Wear goggles or plastic spectacles when using jumper cables or changing car batteries and around chemical sprays, cleaning fluids, darts, pellet and BB guns, power tools, fishing hooks, fireworks (especially bottle rockets), bows and arrows, lawn mowers, hammers, and champagne corks.

□ Wear commercial sunglasses labeled "100% ultraviolet blockage" when exposed to snowfields or bright sunlight.

□ Never look directly at the sun, an eclipse of the sun, or a tanning or arc-welding lamp.

CHAPTER 6

Systemic Diseases

In the diagnostic evaluation of many systemic diseases, the eyes supply critical information. In other cases, the eyes require management directly. Both circumstances may trigger consultation with an ophthalmologist. This chapter lists, in alphabetical order, selected systemic conditions with important ophthalmic manifestations (highlighted in boldface type). Each section also suggests treatment and referral guidelines for the ophthalmic component.

Acne Rosacea

Blepharitis, **keratitis**, and **corneal ulcers** occur in more than 50% of cases, often before or more prominently than skin manifestations. These findings are not specific, but they suggest the diagnosis of acne rosacea when combined with characteristic, if subtle, skin abnormalities.

Treatment and Referral

- Blepharitis: see "Chronic Blepharitis" in Chapter 4.
- Keratitis: see "Keratitis" in Chapter 4.
- Corneal ulcer: refer urgently.

Emergent = immediately. Urgent = within 48 hours. Nonurgent = later than 48 hours.

Acquired Immunodeficiency Syndrome

Retinal cotton-wool spots (Figure 6-1) are present in about 50% of patients who have tested positive for the human immunodeficiency virus (HIV). Although sometimes the first clue, cotton-wool spots are not specific for the acquired immunodeficiency syndrome (AIDS). They indicate only that small retinal precapillary arterioles have become occluded, a phenomenon that occurs in a myriad of conditions. **Kaposi's sarcoma** is a dark red mass that occurs in 25% of HIV-positive patients, sometimes on the eyelids or conjunctiva. It is often mistaken for a stye or subconjunctival hemorrhage. **Cytomegalovirus (CMV) chorioretinitis** occurs in advanced AIDS (Figure 6-2). The diagnosis can be presumed on the basis of the characteristic clinical appearance of hemorrhagic perivascular yellow-white necrosis of the retina.

Treatment and Referral

☐   Retinal cotton-wool spots: no treatment.

☐   Kaposi's sarcoma: no treatment.

☐   CMV chorioretinitis: prescribe intravenous foscarnet or ganciclovir.

Ankylosing Spondylitis

Anterior uveitis occurs in about 33% of patients and may precede rheumatologic symptoms.

Treatment and Referral

☐   See "Anterior Uveitis" in Chapter 4.

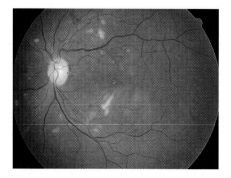

Figure 6-1 Cotton-wool spots. A sign of retinal precapillary arteriolar occlusion and retinal microinfarction. (Courtesy W.K. Kellogg Eye Center, University of Michigan.)

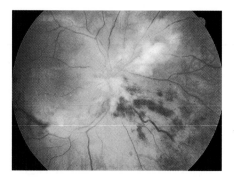

Figure 6-2 Cytomegalovirus chorioretinitis. Occurs in advanced AIDS and other immunocompromised states. (Courtesy W.K. Kellogg Eye Center, University of Michigan.)

Atopic Allergy

Allergic conjunctivitis (conjunctival hyperemia and swelling, stringy discharge, itching, tearing) is usually a component of seasonal allergic upper respiratory tract symptoms, but may be the most prominent and bothersome one. The combination of itching, conjunctival hyperemia, and swelling is distinctive.

Treatment and Referral

☐ See "Allergic Conjunctivitis" in Chapter 4.

Behcet's Disease

About 70% of patients have **uveitis** or **retinal vasculitis** at some time in the course of their illness, often preceding and exceeding other manifestations. Ocular findings are, by themselves, nonspecific.

Treatment and Referral

☐ Anterior uveitis: see "Anterior Uveitis" in Chapter 4.

☐ Posterior uveitis and retinal vasculitis: refer urgently (systemic cytotoxic agents may be of greater benefit than corticosteroids in treatment).

Candidiasis, Systemic

Fungus balls in the retina and vitreous cavity (Figure 6-3) are found in as many as 30% of patients with candidemia consequent to chronic parenteral hemodialysis or hyperalimentation and following severe burns, major surgery (especially gastrointestinal), or long-term antibiotic therapy. Ocular involvement is often asymptomatic at first and may be present even though serial blood cultures are

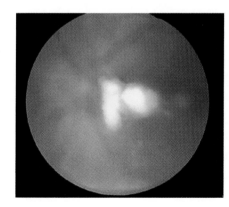

Figure 6-3 Candida vitritis. Fuzzy, yellow-white "fungus balls" obscure the retina. (Courtesy W.K. Kellogg Eye Center, University of Michigan.)

negative. Presumptive diagnosis of systemic candidiasis infection can usually be made by indirect ophthalmoscopy. Vitreous aspiration may provide organisms.

Treatment and Referral

☐   Prescribe intravenous antifungal agents.

Child Abuse, Suspected

Retinal and vitreous hemorrhages (Figure 6-4) may be the only verifiable sign of trauma, especially in "shaken-baby syndrome."

Treatment and Referral

☐   Retinal and vitreous hemorrhages: refer urgently.

Chlamydial Infection

Chlamydial infection presents ocularly as venereally acquired **conjunctivitis** in neonates and adults. In neonates, it is the most common cause of red eye, affecting 2% to 4% of babies. Chlamydial infection is first noticeable from day 2 of life to as late as week 8 and may be indistinguishable from viral or bacterial conjunctivitis. Conjunctivitis may be a clue to other chlamydial infection such as pneumonitis. In adults, it is a chronic low-grade conjunctivitis that is often misdiagnosed as allergic or viral.

Treatment and Referral

☐   See "Chlamydial Conjunctivitis" in Chapter 4 and Table 4-1.

Figure 6-4 Retinal hemorrhages in suspected child abuse. (Courtesy W.K. Kellogg Eye Center, University of Michigan.)

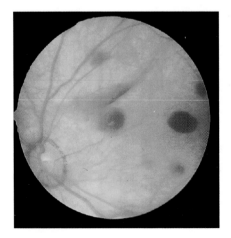

Craniosynostosis

The prevalence of ophthalmic abnormalities is uncertain, but is greater if the characteristic skull or facial deformity is severe. **Papilledema** and **optic atrophy** reflect the effects of chronic increased intracranial pressure on the optic nerves. **Strabismus** may be caused by the orbital deformity.

Treatment and Referral

☐ Papilledema and optic atrophy: refer nonurgently; early decompressive skull surgery by a neurosurgeon may prevent permanent visual loss.

☐ Strabismus: refer nonurgently to an ophthalmologist for possible eye muscle surgery.

Cytomegalovirus Infection

Cytomegalovirus (CMV) infection results in **chorioretinitis.** In infants, infection is acquired prenatally; in adults, it is associated with AIDS or some other immunocompromised state. Adult chorioretinitis is so distinctive that a presumptive diagnosis of systemic CMV infection can be made with the ophthalmoscope (see Figure 6-2).

Treatment and Referral

☐ Prescribe intravenous foscarnet or ganciclovir (halts or reverses chorioretinitis, but if treatment is discontinued, eye disease recurs).

Diabetes Mellitus

Diabetic retinopathy is a common, vision-threatening, and distinctive manifestation of both insulin-dependent and non–insulin-dependent diabetes. Signs of early (nonproliferative) retinopathy include **retinal microaneurysms, hemorrhages,** and **cotton-wool spots.** Nonproliferative diabetic retinopathy causing vision-reducing **macular edema** is present in 12% to 20% of diabetic patients at 15 years after diagnosis. **Retinal neovascularization** and **fibrous proliferation** characterize proliferative diabetic retinopathy, which may produce complete blindness from **vitreous hemorrhage** (see Figure 9-4A) and **retinal detachment.** Proliferative retinopathy is present in 10% to 40% of diabetic patients at 15 years after diagnosis, being more prevalent among those who require insulin. In several large-scale collaborative trials, laser photocoagulation surgery reduced the likelihood of severe visual loss by 50% in certain subgroups. Early diagnosis and treatment of diabetic retinopathy are essential to preserving vision.

Treatment and Referral

- ☐ Tight control of blood sugar markedly reduces the chances of developing retinopathy.
- ☐ Refer patients with diabetes for periodic ophthalmologic examinations based on the age at diagnosis (see the Close-Up "Initial Ophthalmologic Examination of Diabetic Patients" in Chapter 2). Retinal laser photocoagulation surgery is most effective if given before retinal manifestations are severe, usually before patients are visually symptomatic.

Disseminated Intravascular Coagulation

Multifocal choroidal occlusions, causing **outer retinal infarction** and **retinal detachment**, have an unknown prevalence in disseminated intravascular coagulation (DIC) but may be the most verifiable clinical abnormality. Although other conditions may cause these findings, in the proper context they support a diagnosis of DIC.

Treatment and Referral

- ☐ Retinal manifestations: treatment is directed at coagulopathy or the underlying disease.

Down Syndrome

Nystagmus affects about 33% of patients; **strabismus**, 30%; **high myopia and astigmatism**, 25%; **keratoconus**, 15%; and **cataract**, 10%.

Treatment and Referral

- ☐ Refer nonurgently even if no ophthalmic abnormalities are obvious.

Dysproteinemias

Dysproteinemias such as Waldenstrom's macroglobulinemia and multiple myeloma cause numerous ocular disturbances. **Dilated retinal and conjunctival veins**, ascribed to hyperviscosity, have been described in up to 50% of patients. The slow flow may lead to **central retinal vein occlusion** (see Figure 9-12B) or **retinal infarction** (see Figure 9-9), which can cause irreversible visual loss. **Proptosis** is caused by an orbital mass, a very rare finding. **Conjunctival and corneal crystals**, caused by protein deposition, are of uncertain prevalence. **Retinal cotton-wool spots** may occur in some patients.

Treatment and Referral

☐ Central retinal vein occlusion: refer urgently.

☐ Other ophthalmic manifestations: direct treatment at the systemic disease.

Embolic Disease

Emboli (yellow or gray-white) can lodge within retinal arterioles, typically at bifurcations (see Figure 3-6); **ischemic retinal whitening** occurs in cases of arterial obstruction. Patients typically have risk factors for atherosclerotic cardiovascular disease. Sudden, monocular, *persistent* visual loss suggests a total or branch **occlusion of the central retinal artery.** Amaurosis fugax, or *transient* loss of vision (lasting several minutes and then gradually returning to normal), suggests a temporary **embolic obstruction of the central retinal artery.** Like retinal artery occlusion, transient monocular visual loss in patients over 40 years of age is presumed to be thromboembolic from the carotid artery or heart.

Treatment and Referral

☐ Central retinal artery occlusion: see "Acute Persistent Visual Loss" in Chapter 3.

Endocarditis, Bacterial

Ocular findings include **retinal cotton-wool spots, hemorrhages, Roth spots** (white-centered hemorrhages, Figure 6-5), **arterial occlusions, retinal infections** caused by septic microemboli, and **hypersensitivity vasculitis.** The retinal findings represent arterial occlusion and suggest the possibility of emboli. They are not specific for endocarditis and are present only in a minority of patients. Septic emboli may rarely give rise to a **bacterial retinitis** whose manifestations are distinctive.

Figure 6-5 Roth spots (white-centered retinal surface hemorrhages) and a focus of infectious retinitis (white) in bacterial endocarditis. (Courtesy W.K. Kellogg Eye Center, University of Michigan.)

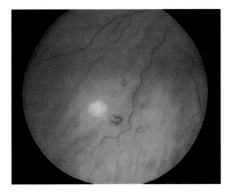

Treatment and Referral

☐ Direct treatment at the systemic disease.

Fibrous Dysplasia

Proptosis and asymmetric facial bone growth characterize fibrous dysplasia. The condition may appear as a monostotic form (involves only one bone) or a polyostotic form (involves many bones), together with endocrine dysfunction. **Optic atrophy** reflects optic nerve compression by bony overgrowth of the optic canal.

Treatment and Referral

☐ Refer nonurgently; surgical decompression of the optic canal may prevent permanent visual loss.

Giant-Cell Arteritis

Ischemic optic neuropathy (see Figure 9-9) and, less commonly, **central retinal artery occlusion** (see Figure 9-12A-1) present as sudden, painless, monocular blindness, occurring in 30% to 50% of patients with giant-cell arteritis, also called *cranial* or *temporal arteritis*. The visual loss caused by an infarction of the optic nerve or retina usually strikes suddenly and irreversibly; only rarely is there a warning symptom of transient visual loss over 1 to 5 days. Most patients have had one or more of the following features: new headache, scalp tenderness, jaw claudication, fever, anorexia, proximal joint and muscle stiffness. The sedimentation rate is usually elevated. However, patients may have no constitutional symptoms and a normal sedimentation rate. Temporal artery biopsy is 95% sensitive to the diagnosis if performed properly.

Treatment and Referral

☐ See "Acute Persistent Visual Loss" in Chapter 3. Prompt and intensive treatment largely prevents blindness in the unaffected eye. Without treatment, the other eye acquires the ischemic optic neuropathy in more than 50% of cases.

Gonococcal Infection

Gonococcal (*Neisseria*) infection is acquired most commonly by neonates from an infected birth canal, although children and adults can also acquire it (Figure 6-6). This infection is the most dangerous cause of **neonatal conjunctivitis**,

Figure 6-6 Gonococcal (*Neisseria*) conjunctivitis in an infant. Marked purulence is distinctive.

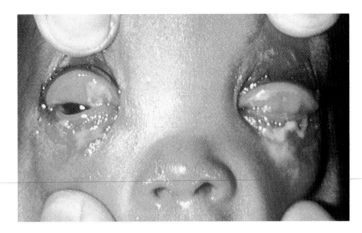

because it often leads to **corneal scarring and perforation** if not treated early. Diagnosed in an estimated 0.6% of babies, gonococcal infection is evident by day 2 or 4 of life as a red eye with copious purulent discharge. Other mucosal surfaces are infected in 16% of cases. A similar infection acquired later in childhood suggests sexual abuse.

Treatment and Referral

☐ See "Bacterial Conjunctivitis" in Chapter 4 and Table 4-1.

Graves' Disease

Ophthalmic effects of Graves' disease (**lid retraction, conjunctival injection, tearing, proptosis, reduced eye movements, strabismus,** and **optic neuropathy**) may cause more symptoms than the systemic effects of the metabolic abnormality (see Figure 4-6). In fact, they often occur in euthyroid patients. External ocular signs may be misdiagnosed as infectious or allergic conjunctivitis or orbital infection or tumor. Optic neuropathy, due to compression of the optic nerve by swollen extraocular muscles, must be treated promptly to prevent permanent visual loss.

Treatment and Referral

☐ Refer if the patient complains of persistent visual loss, pain, or diplopia. Optic neuropathy is treated with systemic corticosteroids, x-irradiation, or surgical removal of the maxillary and ethmoid walls of the orbit. There is no satisfactory treatment for other manifestations in the active phase of the illness. Once the disease is inactive, eye muscle surgery may be undertaken to correct residual ocular misalignment.

Herpes Simplex Infection, Neonatal Form

Herpes simplex infection produces **cutaneous vesicles**, **conjunctivitis**, **keratitis**, and **chorioretinitis** in neonates. The combination of several ophthalmic findings is distinctive in this condition, which is caused by type 2 herpes simplex virus acquired from an infected birth canal. Encephalitis is often present.

Treatment and Referral

☐ Prescribe intravenous acyclovir.

☐ Refer urgently if ocular or periocular manifestations are present. Topical antiherpetic agents such as trifluorothymidine (trifluridine), idoxuridine, or vidarabine are prescribed by the ophthalmologist for anterior ocular manifestations. These agents are used even when keratitis is not present, to prevent eyelid or conjunctival infection from spreading to the cornea, where scarring may cause permanent visual loss. **Caution:** Do not prescribe corticosteroids, because they invite viral replication and contribute to further eye damage.

Herpes Simplex Infection, Primary Form

Primary herpes simplex infection produces **cutaneous vesicles**, **conjunctivitis**, and **keratitis**. The combination of preauricular lymphadenopathy, periocular or facial vesicles, and conjunctival injection is typical. Keratitis is less common than in the recurrent form (see below). Usually an isolated infection of type 1 herpes simplex virus in a healthy patient, the condition may also occur in an immunocompromised host. Slit-lamp biomicroscopy reveals a corneal epithelial defect that often (but not always) has a Christmas-tree–branch (dendritic) configuration. Herpes zoster infection (see below) is the alternative diagnosis; the lack of dermatomal skin involvement weighs against zoster.

Treatment and Referral

☐ Refer urgently; treatment includes topical antiherpetic agents, as for neonatal and recurrent herpes simplex infection.

Herpes Simplex Infection, Recurrent Form

Ocular findings include **conjunctivitis**, **keratitis**, and **uveitis**. Keratitis is usually dendritic (see Figure 1-6B); uveitis is nonspecific. Eyelid skin vesicles may occur, but less commonly than in primary herpes simplex infection. Recurrent outbreaks probably represent reactivation of dormant type 1 virus in trigeminal nerve ganglia. The trigger factors are uncertain.

Treatment and Referral

☐ Refer urgently; treatment includes topical antiherpetic agents, as for neonatal and primary herpes simplex infection. Recurrences are common and require prompt ophthalmologic treatment to prevent visual loss.

Herpes Zoster Infection

Dermatomal configuration of **cutaneous vesicles** involving the first trigeminal dermatome is the diagnostic clue; **keratitis** and **uveitis** are especially likely if vesicles are present on the nose (Hutchinson's sign). The form of keratitis can resemble that caused by herpes simplex.

Treatment and Referral

☐ Cutaneous vesicles: prescribe oral acyclovir 800 mg 5 times daily to reduce the likelihood of keratitis or uveitis.

☐ Keratitis: see "Keratitis" in Chapter 4.

☐ Uveitis: see "Anterior Uveitis" in Chapter 4.

Homocystinuria

Dislocated lenses (usually dislocated inferiorly) occur in 30% of infants with homocystinuria, 80% by age 15. **Large refractive errors** and **glaucoma** may result.

Treatment and Referral

☐ Refer all patients nonurgently, even if asymptomatic.

Hypertension, Acute

Acute hypertension (including that induced by pregnancy) may produce **retinal cotton-wool spots, hard exudates, optic disc edema** (Figure 6-7), **retinal hemorrhages,** and **multifocal choroidal occlusions.** Ophthalmoscopy can help determine whether the elevated blood pressure is causing an ischemic effect on blood vessels and retinal tissue, and, by extension, on cerebral vessels and parenchyma. Optic disc edema is commonly associated with hypertensive encephalopathy.

Treatment and Referral

☐ Cautious lowering of blood pressure is recommended to avoid compromising optic nerve perfusion.

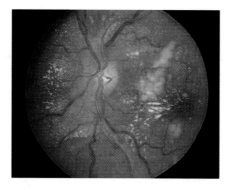

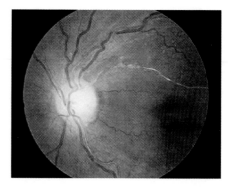

Figure 6-7 Acute hypertensive retinopathy. Note the cotton-wool spots, hard exudates, and optic disc swelling. (Courtesy W.K. Kellogg Eye Center, University of Michigan.)

Figure 6-8 Chronic hypertensive retinopathy. Note the increased light reflections (copper-wiring and silver-wiring) from arterioles and arteriovenous nicking.

Hypertension, Chronic

Ophthalmoscopy can help determine the degree of retinal (and nonocular) arteriolar sclerosis caused by chronic systemic hypertension. Signs include **retinal arteriovenous nicking** and **copper-wire and silver-wire appearance of the arterioles** (Figure 6-8).

Treatment and Referral

☐ Cautious lowering of blood pressure is recommended to avoid compromising optic nerve perfusion.

Hypovitaminosis A

Hypovitaminosis A (malnutrition) produces **conjunctival keratinized spots** (Bitot's spots), **corneal drying** (xerosis), and **corneal scarring**. Ocular findings serve as markers for the degree of malnutrition and increased mortality. Untreated corneal drying leads to corneal perforation and loss of sight.

Treatment and Referral

☐ Direct treatment at the underlying condition.

☐ Treat corneal drying with artificial tears.

Leukemia

Retinal cotton-wool spots, **hemorrhages**, and **Roth spots** (white-centered hemorrhages) reflect the effects of ischemia from anemia and hyperviscosity on blood vessel walls (Figure 6-9). Visual loss may be an early manifestation, but retinal abnormalities may exist without causing visual symptoms.

Treatment and Referral

☐   Direct treatment at the systemic disease.

Lupus Erythematosus, Systemic

Retinal cotton-wool spots, hemorrhages, and **Roth spots** (white-centered hemorrhages) are common when the disease is active, but the exact prevalence is uncertain. These signs are usually asymptomatic and not specific, representing vascular occlusion from one or more of the following mechanisms: immune-complex deposition, antiphospholipid antibody–induced thrombosis, blood dyscrasia, or emboli from nonbacterial endocarditis.

Treatment and Referral

☐   Direct treatment at the systemic disease.

Lysosomal Enzyme Deficiencies

Ocular abnormalities are frequent in lysosomal enzyme deficiencies. They include a **cherry-red** or **gray macula** (Figure 6-10), **pigmentary retinopathy, optic atrophy,** and **corneal opacities** (Table 6-1, "Ophthalmic Manifestations of Lysosomal Enzyme Deficiencies").

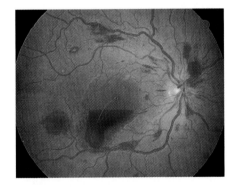

Figure 6-9 Acute leukemia. Retinal and preretinal hemorrhages reflect a low platelet count and low hemoglobin. (Courtesy W.K. Kellogg Eye Center, University of Michigan.)

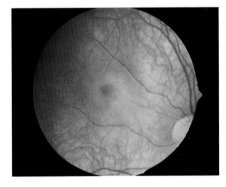

Figure 6-10 Cherry-red spot in Tay-Sachs disease. (Courtesy W.K. Kellogg Eye Center, University of Michigan.)

TABLE 6-1
Ophthalmic Manifestations of Lysosomal Enzyme Deficiencies

Lysosomal Deficiency State	Principal Ocular Findings
Gangliosidoses	
Generalized (GM$_1$, type 1)	Cherry-red macula
Juvenile generalized (GM$_1$, type 2)	Pigmentary retinopathy
Tay-Sachs (GM$_2$, type 1)	Cherry-red macula
Sandoff (GM$_2$, type 2)	Cherry-red macula
Gaucher's disease, type 1	Cherry-red or gray macula
Mucolipidoses	
Types 1 and 2	Cherry-red macula
Type 3	Subtle corneal opacities
Type 4	Corneal clouding, pigmentary retinopathy
Mucopolysaccharidoses	Corneal clouding, pigmentary retinopathy
Niemann-Pick disease	
Type A	Cherry-red macula
Type B	Gray macula
Type C	Vertical-gaze palsy
Metachromatic leukodystrophy	Gray macula, optic atrophy
Multiple sulfatase deficiency	Cherry-red macula, pigmentary retinopathy
Krabbe's disease	Optic atrophy
Fabry's disease	Whorl-like corneal opacities, conjunctival and retinal vessel tortuosity
Farber's disease	Gray macula

Abnormalities may be obvious, as in the corneal clouding of some mucopolysaccharidoses, or subtle, as in the cherry-red or gray macula, pigmentary retinopathy, or corneal whorls.

Treatment and Referral

☐   Direct treatment at the systemic condition.

Marfan's Syndrome

Between 50% and 80% of patients have **dislocated lenses**, usually superiorly (Figure 6-11). The dislocation may cause **glaucoma**, and the lens often becomes opacified, leading to **cataract**. **Retinal detachment** is common, and **large refractive errors** also may result.

Treatment and Referral

☐ Refer all patients nonurgently, even if asymptomatic.

Multiple Sclerosis

Internuclear ophthalmoplegia (deficient adduction), **optic neuropathy**, and **retinal venous sheathing** are present in more than 75% of patients and may be minimally symptomatic. (See "Optic Neuritis" in Chapter 9 for more information.)

Treatment and Referral

☐ Intravenous corticosteroids and subcutaneous beta interferon reduce nonvisual exacerbations. Oral prednisone increases recurrences of optic neuritis.

Myasthenia Gravis

More than 50% of patients have **ptosis** or **ophthalmoplegia** as the presenting sign. Eventually, more than 90% of patients have these signs. Symptoms are often variable and worsened by fatigue. Complete neurologic evaluation with intravenous edrophonium chloride (Tensilon test) is helpful in making the diagnosis.

Figure 6-11 Lens dislocation in Marfan's syndrome. Upward dislocation is typical. Downward dislocation is characteristic in homocystinuria. (Courtesy W.K. Kellogg Eye Center, University of Michigan.)

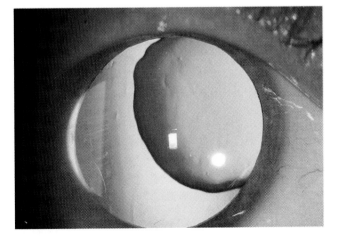

Treatment and Referral

☐ Direct treatment at the systemic disease.

☐ Refer patients with persistent ocular manifestations. In 50% of cases, ocular manifestations are not eliminated with systemic anticholinesterase treatment, so that prisms or occluders may be necessary.

Myotonic Dystrophy

Nearly 100% of patients have a distinctive lens opacity, consisting of multicolored flecks that radiate from the center of the anterior and posterior cortex. This **Christmas-tree cataract** eventually matures into a nonspecific opacity. An uncertain number of patients also have **pigmentary retinopathy**, consisting of ring-like macular hypopigmentation and peripheral retinal salt-and-pepper pigmentation.

Treatment and Referral

☐ There are no treatments for the ophthalmic manifestations, other than cataract extraction.

Neurofibromatosis Type I

Among patients 6 years of age or older, 90% have **iris hamartomas** (Lisch nodules), which are visible by careful slit-lamp examination (Figure 6-12). **Optic nerve/chiasm gliomas**, present in 15%, may cause progressive visual loss. **Plexiform eyelid neurofibromas** and **glaucoma** are less common. When eyelid masses are present, 50% of patients also have glaucoma.

Figure 6-12 Lisch nodules of the iris in neurofibromatosis type I. Nodules appear as tan excrescences on the anterior iris surface. (Courtesy W.K. Kellogg Eye Center, University of Michigan.)

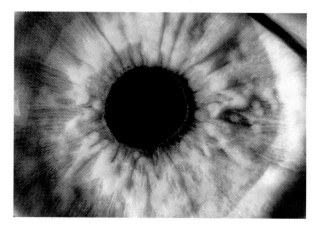

Treatment and Referral

☐ Enlarging optic nerve/chiasm gliomas: refer for radiation or chemotherapy if vision is declining.

☐ Plexiform neurofibromas and glaucoma: refer for surgery.

Pemphigoid, Cicatricial

Cicatricial pemphigoid produces a **chronic, noninfectious conjunctivitis** and **scarring** that lead to severe **drying and scarring of the cornea.** Conjunctival injection precedes scarring and may be misdiagnosed as an infectious condition.

Treatment and Referral

☐ Refer nonurgently; treatment includes artificial tears, systemic corticosteroids, and immunosuppressives, which may arrest or reverse the manifestations.

Pseudoxanthoma Elasticum

Retinal angioid streaks are found in 85% of patients with pseudoxanthoma elasticum, PXE (Figure 6-13). These reddish brown irregular lines, extending radially from the optic nerve head, represent cracks in Bruch's membrane, through which new and fragile choroidal vessels grow into the retina. Most affected patients eventually lose vision from subretinal bleeding. Angioid streaks may also be found less commonly in Ehlers-Danlos syndrome, sickle cell anemia, and Paget's disease.

Treatment and Referral

☐ Refer nonurgently even if asymptomatic. Prophylactic laser photocoagulation surgery reduces the chance of retinal bleeding and visual loss.

☐ Patients are sometimes advised to avoid contact sports because of the risk of retinal hemorrhage.

Figure 6-13 Retinal angioid streaks in pseudoxanthoma elasticum. Subretinal red streaks emanating from the optic disc represent cracks in Bruch's membrane, which separates the retinal pigment epithelium from the choroid. (Courtesy W.K. Kellogg Eye Center, University of Michigan.)

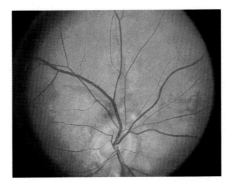

Regional Enteritis

Episcleritis and **uveitis** are present in 10% of patients with regional enteritis, also called *Crohn's disease*. The association between the ocular findings and the enteritis is often overlooked.

Treatment and Referral

☐ See "Episcleritis and Scleritis" and "Anterior Uveitis" in Chapter 4.

Reiter's Syndrome

Conjunctivitis is found in about 30% of patients, together with urethritis and arthritis. **Keratitis** and **uveitis** occur less commonly.

Treatment and Referral

☐ See "Keratitis," "Anterior Uveitis," and "Immunogenic Conjunctivitis" in Chapter 4.

Rheumatoid Arthritis, Adult Form

Dry eye (keratitis sicca) is found in up to 25% of patients. **Sclerokeratitis** is relatively uncommon but important because it is associated with severe systemic vasculitis (Figure 6-14).

Treatment and Referral

☐ Dry eye: prescribe artificial tears; if still symptomatic after several weeks, refer for punctal occlusion.
☐ Sclerokeratitis: see "Episcleritis and Scleritis" in Chapter 4.

Figure 6-14 Sclerokeratitis in adult rheumatoid arthritis. The corneoscleral junction is ulcerated, suggesting the presence of systemic vasculitis.

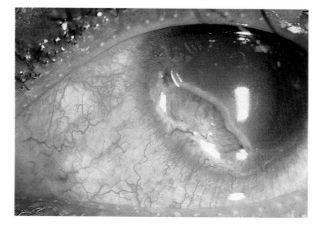

Rheumatoid Arthritis, Juvenile Form

Uveitis occurs in 50% of pauciarticular arthritis patients and much less commonly in polyarticular forms. Uveitis may be asymptomatic and apparent only with slit-lamp biomicroscopy, yet it can lead to **cataract** and **glaucoma** if untreated.

Treatment and Referral

☐   See "Anterior Uveitis" in Chapter 4. Uveitis in this condition is chronic and requires constant monitoring.

Rubella, Congenital

Ocular defects occur in 70% of children whose unimmunized mothers were exposed to rubella during the first 3 months of pregnancy. The defects range from mild to severe and include **microphthalmia, cataract, glaucoma, corneal opacification, uveitis,** and **retinopathy.**

Treatment and Referral

☐   Refer all patients nonurgently.

Sarcoidosis

The eye is affected in 20% to 30% of cases, the third most commonly involved organ (after the lungs and lymph nodes). **Uveitis** accounts for 60% of ocular involvement and is often low-grade and asymptomatic, yet it can eventually cause blindness (Figure 6-15). Results of conjunctival biopsies are positive in 50% of cases when **conjunctival nodules** are seen, but positive in only 5% if the

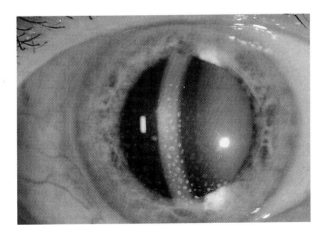

Figure 6-15 Uveitis in sarcoidosis. Small opacities on the inner corneal surface are collections of lymphocytes and macrophages (keratic precipitates), typical of, but not specific to, the chronic, indolent uveitis of sarcoidosis. (Courtesy W.K. Kellogg Eye Center, University of Michigan.)

conjunctiva appears normal. Central nervous system sarcoidosis is present in 30% of cases if **retinal vasculitis** or **choroiditis** is found. **Lacrimal gland enlargement** and **optic nerve/chiasm inflammation** also may occur.

Treatment and Referral

☐ Refer all patients nonurgently even if asymptomatic.

Sickle Cell Disease

Ocular findings are common in SC and S-thal forms, uncommon in SS, and rare in AS (Figure 6-16). Vision-threatening abnormalities include **new retinal blood vessels, retinal and vitreous hemorrhages**, and **retinal detachment**. The patient is generally asymptomatic in the early stages, when laser photocoagulation surgery is most effective in preventing advanced retinopathy. Once proliferative changes have taken place, 12% of patients will lose visual acuity to 20/200 or worse within 8 years. The retinal abnormalities in sickle cell disease occur in the retinal periphery, beyond the view of the direct ophthalmoscope.

Treatment and Referral

☐ Refer all patients with SC and S-thal forms of the disease nonurgently for a baseline ophthalmologic examination and periodic followup examinations. Laser photocoagulation surgery may be employed.

Stevens-Johnson Syndrome

About 50% of patients with Stevens-Johnson syndrome (erythema multiforme) display the conjunctival injection and bullous swelling of **acute conjunctivitis**, which may lead to **scarring** and, in time, **drying of the cornea**.

Figure 6-16 Occlusive vasculopathy in hemoglobin SC (sickle-C) disease. Round, orange lesions (salmon patches) represent peripheral retinal hemorrhages. (Courtesy W.K. Kellogg Eye Center, University of Michigan.)

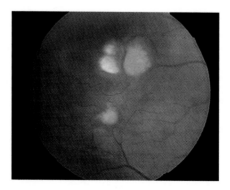

Treatment and Referral

- ☐ Acute conjunctivitis: treatment is of unproven efficacy. Prescribe cold compresses, topical antibiotics, and topical corticosteroids. Refer for possible lysis of conjunctival adhesions.

- ☐ Chronic conjunctivitis: refer all patients nonurgently; treatment is directed at relieving corneal desiccation and preventing abrasion by misdirected eyelashes.

Sturge-Weber Syndrome

Port-wine stain involving the trigeminal dermatome characterizes Sturge-Weber syndrome (encephalotrigeminal angiomatosis). **Glaucoma** is present in 30% of patients, and an even higher percentage if the port-wine stain involves the upper eyelid. Although commonly present from birth, glaucoma may not develop until the second decade. **Choroidal hemangioma** is present in 40% of patients.

Treatment and Referral

- ☐ Refer all patients nonurgently. Glaucoma often requires aggressive management. There is generally no treatment for choroidal hemangioma.

Syphilis

The prevalence of ocular abnormalities in syphilis is unknown. The abnormalities are confined to the secondary and tertiary stages. **Argyll Robertson pupils** are said to be present in more than 50% of tertiary cases. **Keratitis, uveitis**, and **chorioretinitis** may be asymptomatic. **Optic neuritis** may occur.

Treatment and Referral

- ☐ Refer patients who complain of subnormal vision, red eye, or pain nonurgently.

Toxoplasmosis

Toxoplasmosis is usually acquired in utero from mothers infected during pregnancy. Encephalopathy and visceral infection are common, but the eye may be the only evident site of infection. **Chorioretinitis** often reactivates in the teenage years or later. Chorioretinitis is also found in 20% of AIDS patients suspected of having toxoplasmic encephalitis. Toxoplasmosis acquired after birth rarely affects the eye.

Treatment and Referral

☐ Refer nonurgently infants and immunocompromised adults in whom a systemic diagnosis is suspected. Ocular involvement is treated with agents used for the systemic disease: oral pyrimethamine, folinic acid, sulfadiazine, clindamycin, and corticosteroids.

Tuberous Sclerosis

Tuberous sclerosis (Bourneville's disease) produces **retinal astrocytic hamartomas**, ranging in appearance from subtle, flat, translucent plaques to obvious yellow-white "tapioca" mounds on the retinal surface (Figure 6-17). Findings occur in 50% to 80% of patients at any age.

Treatment and Referral

☐ There are no treatments for the ophthalmic findings.

Von Hippel–Lindau Disease

An estimated 75% of patients have one or more **retinal angiomas**, which grow slowly and leak (Figure 6-18). Most often located in the retinal periphery, they cause no visual symptoms until leakage spreads into the macula. If the angiomas are untreated, about 50% of patients eventually become blind in affected eyes.

Treatment and Referral

☐ Refer all patients nonurgently even if asymptomatic. Photocoagulation surgery, cryotherapy, or diathermy is more effective if applied before the lesions become large.

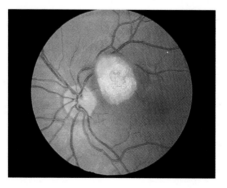

Figure 6-17 Retinal hamartoma (yellow-white) in tuberous sclerosis. (Courtesy W.K. Kellogg Eye Center, University of Michigan.)

Figure 6-18 Retinal angioma in von Hippel–Lindau disease. (**A**) Before and (**B**) after laser photocoagulation surgery. Photocoagulation prevents serious leakage and bleeding, both of which can lead to blindness. (Courtesy W.K. Kellogg Eye Center, University of Michigan.)

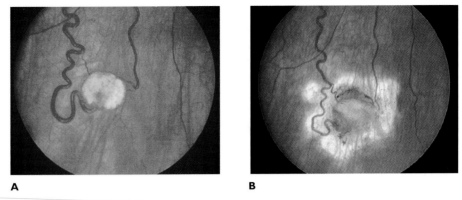

A

B

Wegener's Granulomatosis

Ocular and orbital manifestations can be the first observable signs of disease. They include **chronic conjunctivitis, keratitis, scleritis, sino-orbital inflammation,** and **retinal and optic nerve infarctions.**

Treatment and Referral

☐   Direct treatment at the systemic disease.

Wilson's Disease

A **copper ring** (Kayser-Fleischer ring) in the peripheral cornea is found in 97% of patients with neurologic manifestations of Wilson's disease when examined with the slit-lamp biomicroscope (Figure 6-19). An identical finding is seen in

Figure 6-19 Kayser-Fleischer ring in Wilson's disease. The ring appears greenish brown in the peripheral (limbal) cornea. (Courtesy W.K. Kellogg Eye Center, University of Michigan.)

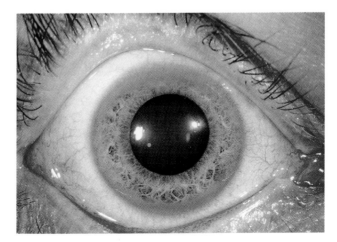

primary biliary cirrhosis. A spoke-like opacity on the anterior and posterior lens capsule (**sunflower cataract**) is present in 15% of patients with Wilson's disease. Corneal and lenticular opacities usually disappear when tissue copper levels are lowered substantially, but remission of ophthalmic signs may not correlate with systemic clinical improvement.

Treatment and Referral

☐   Direct treatment against the abnormal copper metabolism. The Kayser-Fleischer ring often disappears if the copper is successfully removed.

CHAPTER 7

Ophthalmic Medications

This chapter reviews in alphabetical order the ophthalmic medications physicians are most likely to administer or prescribe, as well as the glaucoma agents and anti-inflammatory agents prescribed primarily by ophthalmologists, many of which have important systemic side effects. The Close-Up "Instillation of Medications in the Eye" provides instructions for applying ocular drops and ointments.

Anesthetics

The topical agents used to anesthetize the cornea and conjunctiva are all in the benzocaine family, consisting of the hydrochlorides of proparacaine or tetracaine.

Prototypes

- ☐ Proparacaine hydrochloride 0.5% (many brands)
- ☐ Tetracaine hydrochloride 0.5% (Pontocaine, Anacel)

Mechanism of Action

- ☐ Block trigeminal sensory impulse transmission

Ocular Side Effects

- ☐ Epithelial keratopathy (with habitual use)

CLOSE-UP

INSTILLATION OF MEDICATIONS IN THE EYE

Eyedrops

Improperly instilled eyedrops do not reach the eye. The following technique helps ensure optimal drug delivery.

1. Have the patient recline and tilt the head far back.

2. With the patient looking up, retract the upper lid with the thumb of the hand not holding the eyedropper. Pull down on the skin over the cheekbone with the fingers of the hand that is holding the eyedropper to slightly evert the lower lid (Figure A).

3. Direct the drop at the lower conjunctival cul-de-sac, away from the cornea (see Figure A). **Caution:** If the drop hits the sensitive cornea (Figure B), the patient is likely to blink forcefully and expel the medication.

4. Instill only 1 drop. **Caution:** To avoid contamination, do not allow the tip of the eyedropper to touch any part of the eye or eyelids (Figure C).

5. Immediately after instilling the drop, close the patient's eye and apply digital pressure over the lacrimal sac for 15 to 30 seconds to reduce systemic absorption (Figure D).

6. Wait at least 5 minutes before instilling a second drop, to prevent washout of the first drop from tearing.

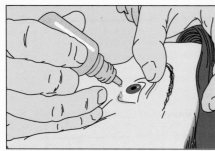

Figure A

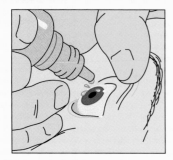

Figure B Wrong way.

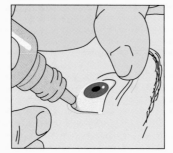

Figure C Wrong way.

Figure D

Systemic Side Effects

☐   None

Comments

Topical anesthetics produce minimal discomfort upon contact with the eye, have an onset of action within 1 minute, and last 10 to 20 minutes; all appear equally effective. Used for diagnostic purposes, they are safe and effective; if used long-term to relieve pain, they may cause blindness. **Caution:** Patients with chronically painful keratopathies may abuse topical anesthetics for pain relief; habitual

Ointments

Ointments are sometimes preferred to eyedrops because they have increased contact time with the ocular surface, providing sustained drug delivery. Ointments also offer a soothing, protective barrier to irritants in the air or on the lid surface and are less likely to be washed away by excessive tearing. The two disadvantages of ointments are that they blur vision and are more difficult for patients to administer correctly.

In applying ointments, proceed as follows:

1. Retract the upper lid and evert the lower lid as for instilling eyedrops, holding the tube of ointment so that the tip of the container is directly over the conjunctival sac (Figure E).

2. Deposit a layer ¼ inch long in the conjunctival cul-de-sac (Figure F). With a twisting motion (rightward for right-handers), detach the ointment from the tip of the container. **Caution:** To prevent contamination and possible inoculation, avoid touching the tip of the container to the eyelid.

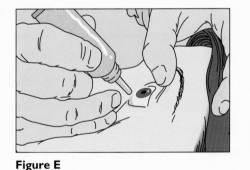

Figure E

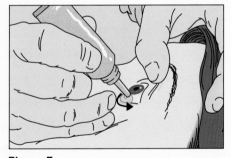

Figure F

use leads to corneal thinning and even perforation. Physicians should never prescribe these drugs.

Anti-infectives

Anti-infective drugs are used to treat ocular adnexal, ocular surface, and intraocular infections. Physicians should be particularly familiar with those used in treating conjunctivitis, blepharitis, and dacryocystitis.

Aminoglycosides

Prototypes

☐ Neomycin (many brands; often combined with polymyxin B, bacitracin, and gramicidin to increase its spectrum of action)

☐ Gentamicin (many brands)

☐ Tobramycin (Tobrex)

Mechanism of Action

☐ Bactericidal

Ocular Side Effects

☐ Contact eyelid and facial dermatitis in about 10% of patients (reversible with topical corticosteroids)

☐ Keratitis with long-term ocular use

Systemic Side Effects

☐ None

Comments

Aminoglycosides are considered the most effective anti-infectives in treating bacterial conjunctivitis, bacterial keratitis, blepharitis, and dacryocystitis. They have rapid action, are broad-spectrum, and are effective against *Pseudomonas* species. However, gentamicin and tobramycin are expensive, and neomycin frequently causes contact dermatitis. Used long-term, they may encourage overgrowth of organisms resistant to many anti-infectives.

Antivirals

Prototypes

☐ Trifluridine 1% (Viroptic)

☐ Vidarabine 3% (Vira-A)

☐ Idoxuridine 0.1% (Herplex, Stoxil, Dendrid)

☐ Acyclovir (Zovirax)

Mechanism of Action

☐ Interfere with viral DNA

Ocular Side Effects

☐ Diffuse epithelial keratopathy

☐ Conjunctival inflammation

☐ Lacrimal punctal stenosis

Systemic Side Effects

□ None

Comments

Trifluridine, vidarabine, and idoxuridine are topical drugs that accelerate the healing of herpes simplex keratitis. All are considered effective, but vidarabine and trifluridine are favored over idoxuridine. Vidarabine is available only as an ointment, trifluridine only as drops, and idoxuridine as both. Acyclovir is available in the United States only for systemic administration, not for topical ocular application. It is administered orally to prevent severe keratitis and uveitis in immune-competent patients with trigeminal herpes zoster, intravenously in immunocompromised patients.

Erythromycin

Prototypes

□ Erythromycin ointment 0.5% (AK-Mycin, Ilotycin)

Mechanism of Action

□ Bacteriostatic

Ocular Side Effects

□ None

Systemic Side Effects

□ None

Comments

Erythromycin is used primarily to treat neonatal inclusion (chlamydial) conjunctivitis, bacterial conjunctivitis, and blepharitis. It is relatively inexpensive and broad-spectrum. Available only as an ointment, it is useful in treating children, who may not cooperate for eyedrop instillation.

Polymyxin B

Prototypes

□ Polymyxin B sulfate (many brands)

Mechanism of Action

□ Bacteriostatic

Ocular Side Effects

□ None

Systemic Side Effects

☐   None

Comments

Polymyxin B is relatively inexpensive, but is always combined with bacitracin, gramicidin, neomycin, trimethoprim, or tetracycline (increasing the cost) to extend its spectrum to gram-positive organisms that cause conjunctivitis or keratitis. When it is combined with neomycin, lid contact allergy is a drawback.

Quinolones

Prototypes

☐   Ciprofloxacin 0.3% (Ciloxan)

☐   Norfloxacin 0.3% (Chibroxin)

Mechanism of Action

☐   Bactericidal

Ocular Side Effects

☐   Crystalline corneal deposits (reversible)

Systemic Side Effects

☐   None

Comments

These potent, broad-spectrum agents, used to treat bacterial conjunctivitis, have poor streptococcal coverage and are expensive.

Sulfa

Prototypes

☐   Sulfacetamide sodium 10% drops and ointment (many brands)

Mechanism of Action

☐   Bacteriostatic

Ocular Side Effects

☐   Rare allergic dermatitis of eyelids

Systemic Side Effects

☐   Extremely rare Stevens-Johnson syndrome in patients previously allergic to systemic sulfa administration

Comments

Sulfacetamide sodium 10% is a good first choice for bacterial conjunctivitis, dacryocystitis, and blepharitis because it is inexpensive, broad-spectrum, and has a low risk of side effects. Do not prescribe if the patient has sulfa allergy.

Tetracycline

Prototypes

☐   Tetracycline hydrochloride 1% (Achromycin, Aureomycin)

Mechanism of Action

☐   Bacteriostatic

Ocular Side Effects

☐   None

Systemic Side Effects

☐   None

Comments

Tetracycline is used primarily in prophylaxis of neonatal conjunctivitis. It is broad-spectrum and especially effective against *Chlamydia,* but is ineffective against *Pseudomonas* species. Systemic effects of topically applied tetracycline are negligible.

Trimethoprim

Prototypes

☐   Trimethoprim–polymyxin B (Polytrim)

Mechanism of Action

☐   Bacteriostatic

Ocular Side Effects

☐   None

Systemic Side Effects

☐   None

Comments

Trimethoprim is an effective, broad-spectrum agent against conjunctival pathogens, but is expensive.

Artificial Tears

Artificial tear preparations are used in patients who have verified tear-deficiency states as occur in Sjogren's syndrome, cicatricial pemphigoid, ocular radiation, and chemical burn. Artificial tears are also prescribed for patients who have normal tear production but have a lid deformity that leaves the eye unprotected from evaporation. In actuality, artificial tears are most often prescribed for patients who complain that their eyes feel dry but have little or no evidence of a dry eye state. Fortunately, these medications have essentially no adverse effects and are relatively inexpensive.

No artificial tear preparation has emerged as a clear favorite for a particular condition. Ophthalmologists may have individual preferences, but they often tell patients to try one or more drugs from each class until an optimal agent is found. For patients with severely dry or exposed eyes, petrolatum-based ointments (usually instilled at bedtime) are an option.

Many patients develop pain and conjunctival inflammation from allergy to the preservatives in artificial tears. For such individuals, artificial tears are available in preservative-free, single-dose vials that are considerably more expensive than standard preparations.

Cellulose Esters

Prototypes
- Hydroxyethylcellulose (many brands)
- Hydroxypropylcellulose (Lacrisert)
- Hydroxypropyl methylcellulose (many brands)
- Methylcellulose (many brands)

Mechanism of Action
- Improve corneal wetting by increasing tear-film viscosity

Ocular Side Effects
- Blurred vision and sticky lids from increased tear viscosity

Systemic Side Effects
- None

Comments
The efficacy of these agents is limited by their short duration of action. They are inexpensive.

Mucomimetics

Prototypes

- ☐ Adapettes
- ☐ Adsorbotears
- ☐ Comfort Drops
- ☐ Dual Wet
- ☐ Hypotears
- ☐ Tears Naturale

Mechanism of Action

- ☐ Increase adherence of aqueous tears to mucin layer that covers corneal surface

Ocular Side Effects

- ☐ None

Systemic Side Effects

- ☐ None

Comments

Mucomimetics have longer duration of action than cellulose esters and polyvinyl alcohol. (All are identified here by brand name because complete generic composition is unrevealed.)

Polyvinyl Alcohol

Prototypes

- ☐ Polyvinyl alcohol (many brands)

Mechanism of Action

- ☐ Increase film-forming property of tears

Ocular Side Effects

- ☐ None

Systemic Side Effects

- ☐ None

Comments

Patients often prefer polyvinyl alcohol over cellulose esters because it is less viscous. This agent is limited by its short duration of action.

Corticosteroids

Although nonsteroidal agents are occasionally used to reduce ocular inflammation, corticosteroids are the mainstay of treatment.

Prototypes

- Prednisolone acetate suspension or sodium phosphate solution 0.125%, 1% (many brands)
- Dexamethasone sodium phosphate suspension, solution 0.1% or ointment 0.05% (many brands)
- Medrysone suspension 1% (HMS)
- Fluorometholone ointment, suspension 0.1% (FML, Flarex, Fluor-Op), 0.25% (FML Forte)

Mechanism of Action

- Reduce inflammation by various means

Ocular Side Effects

- Ocular perforation and intraocular sepsis (by allowing infections and necrotizing inflammations to proceed asymptomatically)
- Elevated intraocular pressure (dose-dependent and usually reversible upon discontinuing the drug; may lead to optic nerve damage if sustained at high levels)

Systemic Side Effects

- None

Comments

All topical ocular corticosteroid preparations are potentially dangerous if used in the following circumstances: an infection has not been excluded; the host is immunocompromised; the globe may be ruptured; ocular trauma involves plants or soil; a red eye has undergone long-term treatment. Combinations of corticosteroids and anti-infectives should be avoided (see the Close-Up "Dangers of Anti-infectives + Corticosteroids").

Decongestants

Ocular decongestants are used to reduce inflammation ascribed to allergy or irritation by pollutants. Two types of topical drugs are sympathomimetic vasoconstrictors and antihistamines, often available in combination. These topical agents may be less effective in relieving allergic manifestations than their systemic counterparts.

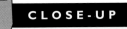

CLOSE-UP

DANGERS OF ANTI-INFECTIVES + CORTICOSTEROIDS

Combinations of anti-infectives and corticosteroids have been prescribed on the basis that the corticosteroid will reduce inflammation while the anti-infective will prevent or eliminate infection. However, infection may still progress after the inflammation has been reduced or eliminated. With the danger signals of redness and pain removed, the patient may not seek attention until the viruses or fungi have produced irrevocable damage. Therefore, combinations of anti-infectives and corticosteroids should not be used.

Antihistamines

Prototypes

☐   Pheniramine maleate 0.3% (many brands)

☐   Antazoline phosphate 0.5% (many brands)

☐   Pyrilamine maleate 0.1% (Prefrin-A)

Mechanism of Action

☐   Block histamine receptors

Ocular Side Effects

☐   None

Systemic Side Effects

☐   None

Comments

Antihistamines are usually combined with vasoconstrictors in prescription and over-the-counter medications used to treat ocular allergy. The addition of topical antihistamines to vasoconstrictors probably increases efficacy but also adds to the cost of the medication.

Vasoconstrictors

Prototypes

☐   Naphazoline hydrochloride 0.05%, 0.1% (many brands)

☐   Tetrahydrozoline hydrochloride 0.05% (many brands)

☐   Phenylephrine hydrochloride 0.12% (many brands)

Mechanism of Action

- Alpha-adrenergic constriction of conjunctival blood vessels

Ocular Side Effects

- Rebound conjunctival hyperemia

Systemic Side Effects

- Hypertension and cardiac arrhythmia (rarely; especially in patients taking monoamine oxidase inhibitors or in those who have labile hypertension)

Comments

These over-the-counter medications are widely used to "get the red out." Although generally harmless, they may mask a serious cause of inflammation, such as keratitis, uveitis, or acute glaucoma. **Caution:** Vasoconstrictors should not be used in combination with systemic monoamine oxidase inhibitors or in patients with labile hypertension.

Glaucoma Agents

Glaucoma agents aim to control intraocular pressure by reducing the production of aqueous humor or by increasing its outflow. Of the five classes of glaucoma drugs, four consist of topically administered agents that work directly on the autonomic nervous system. Despite their local application, absorption into the circulation puts patients at risk for potentially serious systemic side effects. These effects can be reduced by advising patients to maintain finger pressure over the lacrimal sac for 15 to 30 seconds after instilling the eyedrops (see the Close-Up "Instillation of Medications in the Eye"). Carbonic anhydrase inhibitors, the fifth class of glaucoma drugs, differ from the other four classes in that they are administered orally or intravenously. Although they do not affect autonomic function, they cause other important systemic side effects.

Adrenergic Agonists

Prototypes

- Epinephrine 0.25%, 2% (Epifrin, Glaucon)
- Dipivefrin 0.1% (Propine)

Mechanism of Action

- Reduce aqueous humor formation and increase outflow

Ocular Side Effects

- Conjunctival hyperemia
- Black conjunctival deposits (drug metabolites)

Systemic Side Effects

☐ Tachycardia

☐ Premature ventricular contractions

☐ Hypertension

☐ Tremor

☐ Anxiety

Comments

Adrenergic agonists are generally used in conjunction with other glaucoma drugs. They are reasonably well tolerated, but are of relatively low potency and occasionally cause important ocular and systemic side effects.

Beta-Adrenergic Antagonists

Prototypes

☐ Timolol maleate 0.25%, 0.5% (Timoptic)

☐ Betaxolol hydrochloride 0.5% (Betoptic, Betoptic S)

☐ Levobunolol hydrochloride 0.25%, 0.5% (Betagan)

☐ Carteolol hydrochloride 1% (Ocupress)

☐ Metipranolol hydrochloride 0.3% (OptiPranolol)

Mechanism of Action

☐ Decrease aqueous humor secretion from ciliary body

Ocular Side Effects

☐ None that impair function or cause harm

Systemic Side Effects

☐ Bradycardia

☐ Reduced cardiac output and exercise tolerance

☐ Bronchospasm

☐ Hypotension and syncope

☐ Reduced libido

☐ Lethargy and depression

Comments

Because their ocular side effects are unimportant, beta-adrenergic antagonists are the favored agents in treating glaucoma. Nevertheless, their systemic side effects may be dangerous. Between 1978 and 1985, 3000 cases of adverse side effects of timolol were reported to the National Registry of Drug-Induced

Ocular Side Effects. Most involved cardiopulmonary function; 32 were associated with fatalities. While the overall incidence of systemic side effects is uncertain, caution is especially warranted in elderly patients and in patients with cardiopulmonary disease. **Caution:** Effects may be additive and especially harmful in patients who are treated simultaneously with systemic and topical beta-adrenergic drugs.

Carbonic Anhydrase Inhibitors

Prototypes
☐ Acetazolamide (Diamox): tablets 125 mg, 250 mg; capsules 500 mg; also available as parenteral formulation

Mechanism of Action
☐ Decrease aqueous humor secretion by reducing levels of bicarbonate in ciliary processes

Ocular Side Effects
☐ None

Systemic Side Effects
☐ Stevens-Johnson syndrome (erythema multiforme) and blood dyscrasias (idiosyncratic allergic reactions)
☐ Renal stones (associated with long-term therapy; advise patients to avoid dehydration)
☐ Tingling of hands and feet
☐ Nausea
☐ Abnormal taste sensation (dysgeusia)
☐ Anorexia
☐ Lassitude
☐ Loss of libido
☐ Impotence
☐ Systemic acidosis

Comments
Carbonic anhydrase inhibitors (CAIs) are important second- or third-line agents in glaucoma treatment. Some of their systemic side effects are merely unpleasant; others are dangerous. Stevens-Johnson syndrome is especially prevalent among patients who are allergic to sulfa drugs. Blood dyscrasias, particularly aplastic anemia, generally occur within the first 6 months of drug use and tend to be reversed as soon as therapy is stopped. Between 1972 and 1984, 79 allergic reac-

tions to CAIs were reported to the National Registry of Drug-Induced Ocular Side Effects; one third were fatal.

During the first 2 weeks of CAI therapy, patients tend to develop systemic acidosis secondary to potassium and bicarbonate diuresis. These effects are self-limited and are usually not dangerous unless a patient is already potassium-depleted from either thiazide use or renal disease.

Apart from renal stones, the remaining side effects listed are usually mild enough to be tolerated. Patients may begin to complain of the systemic symptoms long after the CAIs were started. The symptoms may often be attenuated by supplemental potassium and calcium.

Cholinergic Agonists

Prototypes
- Pilocarpine hydrochloride and nitrate (many brands)

Mechanism of Action
- Increase aqueous humor outflow

Ocular Side Effects
- Pupillary constriction
- Conjunctival injection
- Brow ache or headache and, in younger patients, ciliary spasm causing reversible myopia

Systemic Side Effects
- Rare when used in proper dosage (4 times a day)
- With overdose (1 drop per hour), may produce abdominal cramping, vomiting, diarrhea, diaphoresis, bronchospasm, unstable blood pressure

Comments
Pilocarpine is inexpensive and effective, but ocular side effects limit its use.

Cholinesterase Inhibitors

Prototypes
- Echothiophate iodide 0.03%, 0.06%, 0.125%, 0.25% (Phospholine Iodide, Echodide)

Mechanism of Action
- Increase aqueous humor outflow

Ocular Side Effects

☐ Marked pupillary constriction

☐ Marked conjunctival hyperemia

☐ Cataract (only after long-term use)

Systemic Side Effects

☐ Abdominal cramping

☐ Vomiting

☐ Diarrhea

☐ Diaphoresis

☐ Bronchospasm

☐ Unstable blood pressure

☐ Prolonged apnea after succinylcholine use in general anesthesia

Comments

Echothiophate iodide is used uncommonly because of its numerous side effects. In view of the apnea problem, patients taking cholinesterase inhibitors should discontinue them at least 2 weeks before undergoing general anesthesia. The drug is also used to treat a form of accommodative esotropia in children.

Mydriatics and Cycloplegics

Topical parasympatholytic agents paralyze the iris sphincter (mydriasis) and the ciliary muscle (cycloplegia). Mydriasis is used to obtain an improved view of the lens, vitreous, and optic fundus. Cycloplegia is used to reduce painful reactive ciliary-muscle spasm in keratitis or uveitis and to suspend accommodation for a more optimal refraction, especially in children.

Topical sympathomimetic agents produce only moderate mydriasis and no cycloplegia.

Parasympatholytics

Prototypes

☐ Tropicamide 0.5%, 1% (Mydriacyl, Tropicacyl)

☐ Cyclopentolate hydrochloride 0.5%, 1%, 2% (Cyclogyl, AK-Pentolate)

☐ Homatropine hydrobromide 2%, 5% (Homatrocel, Isopto Homatropine)

☐ Scopolamine 0.25% (Isopto Hyoscine, Mydramide)

☐ Atropine sulfate 0.5%, 1%, 2%, 3% (many brands)

Mechanism of Action

☐ Block muscarinic receptors of iris sphincter and ciliary muscle

Ocular Side Effects

☐ Temporary loss of accommodation

☐ Temporary photophobia from enlarged pupil

☐ Rare contact dermatitis of eyelids (short-lived; reversible with topical corticosteroid)

☐ Acute angle-closure glaucoma in patients with anatomically narrow anterior chamber angles (very rare; see "Acute Angle-Closure Glaucoma" in Chapter 4 and "Glaucoma" in Chapter 9)

Systemic Side Effects

☐ Fever, skin flush, tachycardia, confusion (predominantly in children treated with atropine or cyclopentolate)

☐ Seizures (very rare; in children with poorly controlled epilepsy)

Comments

Tropicamide is the most commonly used agent for ophthalmoscopy and refraction because of its brief duration of action (4 to 6 hours). Cyclopentolate and atropine are used by ophthalmologists to obtain more complete cycloplegia for refraction in children with strabismus and in treating uveitis. (Cyclomidril, containing cyclopentolate 0.2% and phenylephrine 0.1%, is ideal for infants, with a duration of action of 4 to 6 hours.) The Close-Up "Parasympatholytics for Mydriasis and Cycloplegia" compares the duration of action of the various agents. **Caution:** Do not use atropine for cycloplegia because of its extremely prolonged paralysis of accommodation (1 to 2 weeks).

CLOSE-UP

PARASYMPATHOLYTICS FOR MYDRIASIS AND CYCLOPLEGIA

Agent	Duration of Action
Tropicamide	4 to 6 hours
Cyclopentolate	12 to 24 hours
Homatropine	1 to 3 days
Scopolamine	4 to 7 days
Atropine	1 to 2 weeks

Sympathomimetics

Prototypes

☐ Phenylephrine 2.5%, 10% (many brands)

Mechanism of Action

☐ Stimulate iris dilator muscle

Ocular Side Effects

☐ None

Systemic Side Effects

☐ Phenylephrine 2.5%: none

☐ Phenylephrine 10%: rare blood pressure elevation, cardiac arrhythmia, myocardial infarction

Comments

Phenylephrine 2.5% is very useful to improve the view of the fundus for ophthalmoscopy. Its duration of action is only 1 to 2 hours, and the risk of precipitating angle-closure glaucoma is negligible. Ophthalmologists use this agent primarily as an adjuvant to a parasympatholytic agent (tropicamide or cyclopentolate) when wide mydriasis is desired for complete ophthalmoscopy. **Caution:** Phenylephrine 10% should not be used because it may cause a severe rise in blood pressure, ventricular arrhythmia, and myocardial infarction, especially among patients being treated with systemic beta-blockers.

CHAPTER 8

Systemic Medications

A number of systemically administered agents produce ocular side effects; most are reversible, but some may result in permanent visual loss. In alphabetical order, this chapter presents common systemic medications that have important effects on the visual system. Recommendations are made for managing these ocular side effects.

Amiodarone

Brand name: Cordarone

Nearly all patients treated with conventional doses will develop keratopathy, which takes the form of corneal epithelial whorls visible only with the slit lamp (Figure 8-1). The sign is generally reversible when treatment is stopped. Less than 10% of patients are symptomatic.

Ocular Symptoms and Signs

☐ Halos

☐ Blurred vision (usually very mild)

☐ Corneal epithelial whorls (visible on slit-lamp biomicroscopy)

☐ Optic neuropathy

Treatment and Referral

☐ Discontinue medication, if possible, in rare symptomatic patients.

☐ Refer patients who complain of subnormal vision.

Figure 8-1 Amiodarone keratopathy. Note the brown whorls centered in the inferior portion of the cornea. (Courtesy W.K. Kellogg Eye Center, University of Michigan.)

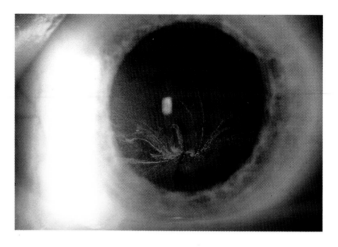

Anticholinergics

Patients under age 50 are at risk for loss of accommodation. In patients over 50, accommodation is already deficient from normal aging so that the effect of an anticholinergic is negligible.

Patients who have an anatomically narrow anterior chamber angle are at risk for angle-closure glaucoma following the slight pupillary dilation caused by systemically administered anticholinergics. Because a shallow anterior chamber is a rare anatomic variant that is difficult to identify and because the incidence of this side effect is so low, it is not reasonable to try to identify patients at risk. Contrary to the information provided in the package inserts of anticholinergic agents, patients with open-angle glaucoma (the most common form) are *not* at risk for angle-closure glaucoma.

Ocular Symptoms and Signs

☐ Loss of accommodation: reduced near visual acuity

☐ Angle-closure glaucoma: visual loss, periocular pain, ciliary flush (perilimbal conjunctival hyperemia), cloudy cornea, elevated intraocular pressure

Treatment and Referral

☐ Warn patients under age 50 of the risk of loss of accommodation. If the medication must be continued, perform a near visual acuity examination and, if the result is subnormal, refer for refraction.

☐ If angle-closure glaucoma is suspected, refer emergently to an ophthalmologist.

Cis-Platinum

Brand name: Platinol

Women over age 50 maintained on very high doses (200 mg/m²/day) are at risk for retinopathy, optic neuropathy, and visual cortex damage.

Ocular Symptoms and Signs

☐ Loss of visual acuity

☐ Loss of color vision

☐ Optic disc edema

☐ Retrobulbar neuritis

☐ Cortical blindness

Treatment and Referral

☐ Refer if the patient complains of visual acuity or color vision loss. When a side effect is suspected, discontinue the drug, if possible; the dose limit for reversibility is not well documented.

Corticosteroids

Among patients maintained on doses equivalent to prednisone 15 mg/day for 1 year or longer, about 25% develop significant cataracts (Figure 8-2); the amount of the cumulative dose appears to be more critical than the amount of the daily dose. Patients are also at risk for developing glaucoma with an unknown frequency. Children are at risk for developing pseudotumor cerebri, especially if the dosage is abruptly decreased after long-term administration.

Figure 8-2 Corticosteroid cataract. The gray opacity is seen against the orange light reflected from the retina. (Courtesy W.K. Kellogg Eye Center, University of Michigan.)

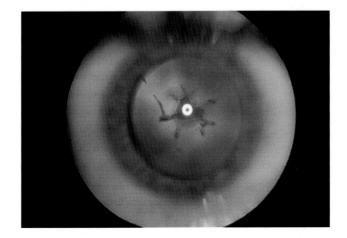

Ocular Symptoms and Signs

- Cataract: subnormal visual acuity, lens opacification
- Glaucoma: elevated intraocular pressure; rarely, glaucomatous optic nerve cupping and visual field loss
- Pseudotumor cerebri: headache, transient visual loss, swollen optic disc, visual field loss

Treatment and Referral

- Cataract: perform periodic visual acuity screening; if acuity is declining, refer for ophthalmologic examination; cataract stops growing if therapy is withdrawn or substantially reduced, but does not regress.
- Glaucoma: refer for monitoring of intraocular pressure every 6 months; intraocular pressure generally normalizes when therapy is withdrawn.
- Pseudotumor cerebri: refer to an ophthalmologist; findings are generally reversible if the condition is discovered early enough.

Cytosine Arabinoside

Patients taking the drug at high intravenous doses (3 g/m^2 every 12 hours for 6 days) are at risk for developing keratitis.

Ocular Symptoms and Signs

- Photophobia, pain, and blurred vision after 5 to 7 days of treatment
- Multifocal corneal epithelial breakdown (punctate fluorescein staining) on slit-lamp biomicroscopy

Treatment and Referral

- Treat prophylactically with topical prednisolone phosphate 1% 4 times daily to markedly reduce this side effect.
- Refer to an ophthalmologist if symptoms persist beyond 1 week or are worsening.

Deferoxamine Mesylate

Brand name: Desferal

Some patients develop retinopathy or optic neuropathy (Figure 8-3). Prevalence and relationship to dose are uncertain. Ophthalmic toxicity may appear acutely and immediately after treatment or subacutely and months after treatment. Symptoms precede signs, especially if toxicity is immediate. Toxicity is at least partially reversible when the drug is withdrawn.

Figure 8-3 Deferoxamine retinal toxicity. The retina has a speckled (salt-and-pepper) appearance. Fine pigment clumps are visible around the fovea. These findings may also be caused by other toxins (thioridazine), infections (rubella, syphilis), and inherited retinal dystrophies. (Courtesy W.K. Kellogg Eye Center, University of Michigan.)

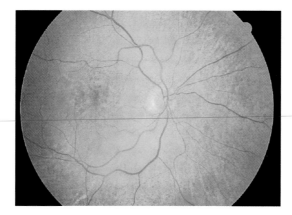

Ocular Symptoms and Signs

☐ Loss of color vision

☐ Loss of visual acuity

☐ Loss of visual field

☐ Macular and peripheral retinal pigment abnormalities

Treatment and Referral

☐ Perform a baseline ophthalmic screening examination. If acuity is subnormal, refer for ophthalmologic examination.

☐ Test visual acuity every 3 months while the patient is taking the drug. Refer for ophthalmologic examination if the medication must be continued beyond 6 months or if symptoms and signs suggest new visual loss.

☐ Withdraw the drug if toxicity is documented.

Digoxin

Brand name: Lanoxin

About 25% of patients whose digoxin levels are in the moderately toxic range develop retinopathy. At high enough doses, all patients develop symptoms and signs of retinal toxicity.

Ocular Symptoms and Signs

☐ Snowy, flickering, or yellowish orange vision (xanthopsia)

Treatment and Referral

☐ Adjust the dose to the therapeutic range; the effects resolve when digoxin levels are lowered.

Ethambutol Hydrochloride

Brand name: Myambutol

Optic neuropathy can develop in patients maintained on daily doses in excess of 15 mg/day or those taking lower doses who have renal failure. Visual loss is reversible only if detected early. Further decline after discontinuing the drug is rare.

Ocular Symptoms and Signs

- Loss of color vision
- Loss of visual acuity
- Loss of visual field

Treatment and Referral

- Perform a baseline ophthalmic screening examination before treatment.
- Test visual acuity every 6 months thereafter.
- If declining visual acuity is documented, discontinue the drug promptly and refer for ophthalmologic examination.

Hydroxychloroquine Sulfate

Brand name: Plaquenil

Patients maintained on daily doses above 400 mg/day for 1 year or more are at risk for retinopathy (Figure 8-4). Even at such dosages, prevalence is low and, for that reason, management is uncertain. Visual deficits are generally not reversible, but further decline is rare once the drug is stopped.

Ocular Symptoms and Signs

- Loss of color vision
- Loss of visual field
- Loss of visual acuity
- Atrophy of the retina surrounding the fovea (bull's-eye lesion)

Treatment and Referral

- Perform a baseline ophthalmic screening examination before treatment. If acuity is subnormal, refer for ophthalmologic examination.
- Test visual acuity every 6 months.

Figure 8-4 Hydroxychloroquine toxicity. A bull's-eye maculopathy reflects atrophy of the perifoveal retinal pigment epithelium.

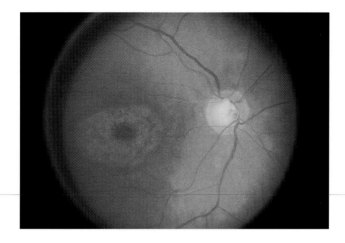

□   If the patient complains of reduced color vision, visual field, or visual acuity, discontinue the drug immediately and refer for ophthalmologic examination.

Isoniazid

Brand name: INH

Optic neuropathy may occur in patients maintained on more than the recommended daily dose: adults, 5 mg/kg; children, 10 to 20 mg/kg. Drug effects may be synergistic with ethambutol. Visual loss is reversible only if detected early. Further decline after discontinuing the drug is rare.

Ocular Symptoms and Signs

□   Loss of color vision

□   Loss of visual acuity

□   Loss of visual field

Treatment and Referral

□   Perform a baseline ophthalmic screening examination.

□   Test visual acuity every 6 months thereafter.

□   If declining visual acuity is documented, discontinue the drug promptly and refer for ophthalmologic examination.

Figure 8-5 Isotretinoin toxicity. The papilledema reflects increased intracranial pressure due to impaired drainage of cerebrospinal fluid. (Courtesy W.K. Kellogg Eye Center, University of Michigan.)

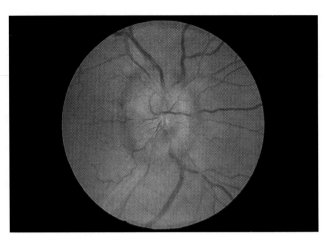

Isotretinoin

Brand name: Accutane

Pseudotumor cerebri is an idiosyncratic rather than a dose-related phenomenon (Figure 8-5). Symptoms and signs may occur within days of starting therapy. They are generally reversible if the condition is discovered early enough.

Ocular Symptoms and Signs

☐   Headache

☐   Transient visual loss

☐   Swollen optic disc

☐   Visual field loss

Treatment and Referral

☐   Refer for ophthalmologic evaluation if the patient complains of transient or permanent visual loss.

☐   Discontinue the medication promptly if pseudotumor cerebri is diagnosed.

Phenytoin and Carbamazepine

Brand name for phenytoin: Dilantin
Brand name for carbamazepine: Tegretol

Patients whose drug levels are in moderately toxic ranges may experience vestibulocerebellar toxicity. The symptoms resolve when serum levels fall to the therapeutic range.

Ocular Symptoms and Signs

- Diplopia
- Blurred vision (secondary to unstable ocular fixation)
- Nystagmus (secondary to interruption of eccentric gaze-holding mechanisms) is not necessarily a sign of drug toxicity, often occurring even at the upper limits of the recommended serum levels

Treatment and Referral

- Adjust the dose downward, if possible, to minimize the symptoms.

Tamoxifen Citrate

Brand name: Nolvadex

Patients are at risk for retinopathy if they are maintained on very high doses (120 mg twice daily) and after a cumulative dose of at least 100 g. However, some cases have also been reported among patients ingesting normal doses (20 mg/day) after a total of 7 g.

Ocular Symptoms and Signs

- Loss of visual acuity
- Cystoid macular edema
- Perimacular crystalline deposits

Treatment and Referral

- Perform a baseline visual acuity examination if treatment with high doses is anticipated.
- Test visual acuity every 6 months thereafter.
- If visual acuity is declining or the patient complains that vision is failing, discontinue or reduce the dose of the medication and obtain ophthalmologic consultation. Visual acuity generally returns to normal within months, but retinal deposits remain.

Thioridazine

Brand name: Mellaril

Patients are at risk for retinopathy if maintained on doses above 800 mg/day. Visual loss is irreversible, and further visual loss may occur despite discontinuing the drug.

Ocular Symptoms and Signs

☐ Brownish discoloration of vision

☐ Reduced visual acuity

☐ Constricted peripheral visual fields

☐ Can also be associated with pigment mottling of the macula and retinal periphery (pigmentary retinopathy)

Treatment and Referral

☐ Perform a baseline ophthalmic screening examination.

☐ Test visual acuity every 6 months in patients taking high doses.

☐ Advise the patient to report discolored or blurred vision or failing night vision.

☐ If declining visual acuity is documented, discontinue the drug promptly and refer for ophthalmologic examination.

Vincristine

Patients on vincristine therapy may experience upper lid ptosis and cranial nerve VI palsy. Toxicity is dose-related, occurring after a mean total dose of 17.7 mg over a 10-week period.

Ocular Symptoms and Signs

☐ Ptosis

☐ Diplopia

☐ Abduction deficits

Treatment and Referral

☐ Perform an ophthalmic external and motility examination if the patient complains of ptosis or diplopia.

☐ Discontinue the drug, if possible. Resolution occurs in 90% of patients, on average 11 weeks after the drug is stopped; the dose limit for reversibility is not well documented.

CHAPTER 9

Principal Conditions

This chapter presents in alphabetical order an overview of 15 of the most important ophthalmic conditions, including their prevalence and clinical significance, diagnosis, and management. The main points for each entity are distilled in the "At a Glance" feature for quick review.

Age-Related Macular Degeneration

AT A GLANCE

☐ Age-related macular degeneration (ARMD), an idiopathic disorder of senescence, is the leading cause of blindness in the older-age population of the United States.

☐ Laser surgery may reduce the risk of severe vision loss in some patients.

☐ Early detection is critical because laser surgery is not effective in advanced cases.

☐ Patients who cannot be helped by laser surgery should be encouraged to make use of optical devices and rehabilitative services.

Age-related macular degeneration (ARMD), formerly known as *senile macular degeneration,* is a slowly progressive, binocular loss of central vision owing to deterioration of the retinal pigment epithelium in the macula. Unlike presbyopia, ARMD is not an inevitable consequence of growing older. This disease is

Figure 9-1 Age-related macular degeneration. (**A**) The yellow deposits called *drusen* indicate malfunction of the retinal pigment epithelium. (**B**) Bleeding under the macula from a subretinal neovascular membrane. (**C**) Fluorescein angiography highlights a neovascular membrane (white frond). (**D**) Laser photocoagulation surgery obliterates the neovascular membrane and leaves an area of yellow-white chorioretinal atrophy. (Courtesy W.K. Kellogg Eye Center, University of Michigan.)

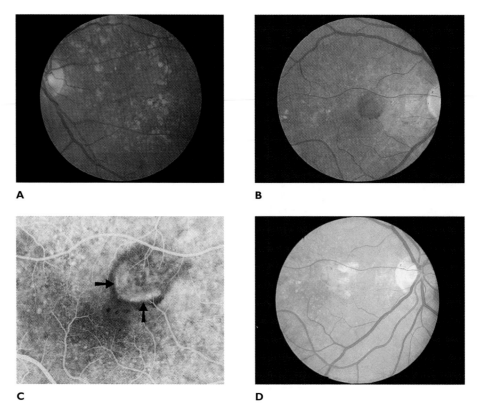

A   B

C   D

of unknown cause; no risk factors or effective preventive measures have been identified.

Prevalence and Clinical Significance

ARMD is the leading cause of legal blindness in adults over age 50. Among individuals aged over 65 years, 2.2% are blind in one eye from this disease. Early diagnosis is important because, in some patients, laser surgery is effective in retarding visual loss.

Diagnosis

The first ophthalmoscopic manifestations of ARMD are drusen, small yellow-white deposits underneath the retina that do not affect vision (Figure 9-1A). In patients destined to develop ARMD, the drusen become confluent and the overlying retinal pigment epithelium becomes atrophic. Central vision is gradually lost.

In an estimated 10% of patients with ARMD, blood vessels from the choroid burrow and bleed into the retina, disrupting its architecture and evoking scar formation (Figure 9-1B). This late development in a small fraction of patients with ARMD causes a sudden, marked fall in visual acuity. In some patients who

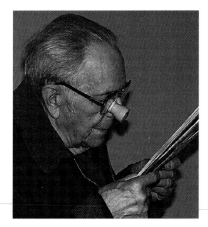

Figure 9-2 Optical devices for patients with ARMD. Some visually impaired patients use a telemicroscope to magnify reading matter. (Courtesy W.K. Kellogg Eye Center, University of Michigan.)

develop these neovascular membranes, visual loss can be retarded by laser surgery.

Management

National collaborative studies have established that laser photocoagulation surgery of errant subretinal blood vessels can significantly arrest the decline in vision. Laser surgery is effective only if the macula has not yet become grossly deformed. Screening for treatable ARMD requires ophthalmoscopy with the assistance of the slit-lamp biomicroscope. Fluorescein angiography may also be necessary to determine whether the condition is treatable (Figure 9-1C). Accordingly, patients identified as having early ARMD should have periodic ophthalmologic examinations.

If the ophthalmologist detects early signs of ARMD with features that are not yet treatable, patients are usually given an Amsler grid (a grid of black lines against a white background) for periodic home self-examination and asked to report if the lines suddenly appear bent, distorted, or missing, which may indicate an appropriate time for treatment. Timely laser photocoagulation surgery may arrest, and sometimes reverse, visual loss (Figure 9-1D).

Patients can be reassured that even though ARMD may cause them to lose reading vision, they will not lose peripheral vision. They should be encouraged to avail themselves of special optical devices and coping strategies for the visually impaired (Figure 9-2; see also the Close-Up "Rehabilitation for the Visually Impaired").

Amblyopia

AT A GLANCE

☐ Amblyopia is a common and often reversible cause of subnormal vision in children, usually affecting only one eye.

☐ Amblyopia arises from strabismus, unequal refractive errors in the two eyes (anisometropia), corneal or lens opacity, or ptosis.

☐ Treatment for amblyopia includes eliminating the predisposing conditions and patching the nonamblyopic eye. Success depends on early detection, elimination of predisposing conditions, and continuity of care.

Amblyopia is reduced vision beginning in early childhood as the result of either suppression of a retinal image or visual deprivation. In physiologic terms, amblyopia represents a failure of visual connections owing to disuse.

Suppression of a retinal image occurs when the eyes are out of alignment (strabismus). To avoid the confusion of seeing the same image in two different locations in space, the brain suppresses the image seen by the deviating eye.

REHABILITATION FOR THE VISUALLY IMPAIRED

Optical Low-Vision Devices

The optimal device depends on the type and degree of visual impairment, the visual task, and personal preference, which can be determined by trying a variety of devices. Five main kinds are available, all providing magnification:

- Magnifying eyeglasses
- Hand magnifiers
- Stand magnifiers
- Telescopes
- Closed-circuit television

Nonoptical Low-Vision Devices

These devices include special lights, large-print reading material, high-contrast watch faces, machines that "talk," and computers that read printed material. They are available through low-vision centers.

Rehabilitation Programs

These include mobility training, redesigning the home environment, Braille instruction, and psychotherapy. Such intensive training is often offered through state or federal (Veterans Administration) rehabilitation programs. The following agencies can provide further information:

- National Association for
  the Visually Handicapped
  22 West 21st Street
  New York, NY 10010
  (212) 889-3141
- The Lighthouse
  800 2nd Avenue
  New York, NY 10017
  1-800-334-5497

- National Library Service for the
  Blind and Physically Handicapped
  Library of Congress
  Washington, DC 20542
  1-800-424-8567
- State commissions for the blind

Visual deprivation occurs when one or both eyes fail to receive well-formed images. Amblyopia occurs in an eye that has a high uncorrected refractive error relative to the other eye (anisometropia), one with a corneal or lens opacity, or one that has ptosis. Low birth weight and parental history of amblyopia or strabismus are contributing risk factors.

Prevalence and Clinical Significance

Amblyopia is the cause of subnormal vision in about 2% of the United States population. If the unaffected eye maintains normal sight, amblyopia limits depth perception. But if another malady later claims the vision of the unaffected eye, the patient's sight will be impaired, as the amblyopia may not be reversible. If amblyopia is recognized at an early stage, it may often be reversed, particularly if the visual system is still immature, that is, before age 9.

Diagnosis

Amblyopia causes no clinically observable structural abnormalities or distinctive signs. Therefore, it is diagnosed by excluding other causes of subnormal vision and by finding one or more of the settings for amblyopia: strabismus, anisometropia, corneal or lenticular opacities, ptosis.

Management

Reversing amblyopia depends on early detection, eliminating predisposing factors, and patching the normal eye to force the patient to use the amblyopic eye. In patients with congenital cataract, keratopathy, or ptosis, surgical correction before 3 months of age is critical to restoring adequate vision. Because amblyopia often recurs, patients require persistent followup. The vulnerable period for developing amblyopia and the potential for restoring normal vision ends at approximately age 9; until that time, the general physician and the ophthalmologist should collaborate in maintaining close rapport with the patient's family to secure regular eye examinations.

Cataract

AT A GLANCE

☐ Cataract is the most common cause of visual loss in the elderly. It causes a diminished red reflex most accurately observed by slit-lamp biomicroscopy through widely dilated pupils.

☐ Surgical removal usually results in excellent visual outcome if cataract is the sole cause of visual loss. Postoperative optical rehabilitation includes intraocular lenses (implants), contact lenses, or eyeglasses.

☐ Nd:YAG laser capsulotomy usually restores vision if the posterior lens capsule has opacified (50% of patients) months to years after cataract extraction.

A cataract is an opacity in the normally transparent focusing lens of the eye that, as it becomes denser, interferes with clear sight. The most common cause is aging; less common causes are intraocular diseases, trauma, medications, and metabolic, endocrine, or congenital abnormalities.

Prevalence and Clinical Significance

Cataract is the most common cause of visual loss in adults. By age 65, more than 90% of all people have cataracts. More than 1 million cataract extractions are performed yearly in the United States.

Cataracts may develop at any age, even in the neonatal period, when early extraction is essential to prevent amblyopia. For this reason, it is important to screen for red fundus reflexes in the neonate and infant.

Diagnosis

An advanced cataract appears as a diminished red reflex through the ophthalmoscope. The ophthalmoscope beam must be aimed perfectly through small pupils to avoid the false impression of a diminished red reflex. Because most vision-impairing cataracts are not completely opaque and may not noticeably interfere with the red reflex, a better diagnostic method is to use the slit-lamp biomicroscope with the patient's pupils widely dilated.

Management

The only method of treating a cataract is surgical removal. Surgery may be deferred until decreased vision interferes with the patient's ability to perform routine activities, except in the following circumstances:

- In neonates, in whom assessment of vision is difficult and in whom visual deprivation may rapidly lead to irreversible amblyopia

- When the cataract interferes with the diagnosis or treatment of other ocular diseases, such as diabetic retinopathy or a potential intraocular malignancy

- When the cataract causes other eye diseases, such as uveitis or glaucoma

In adults, most cataract surgery is performed under local anesthesia as an outpatient procedure. Formerly, the most common practice was to remove the lens and its surrounding capsule (intracapsular extraction). The current technique is to remove only the lens and the anterior capsule (extracapsular extraction), leaving the posterior capsule as a shield against forward displacement of the vitreous and as a support for an intraocular lens.

Phacoemulsification is a method of extracapsular extraction using a high-frequency ultrasound device to fragment the hard nucleus of the lens into smaller particles and then aspirate them. This method enables the surgeon to remove the cataract through a small incision.

When the cataract is removed, the eye is called *aphakic* and optical power must be restored in one of three ways: an intraocular lens, an eyeglass lens, or a contact lens.

Intraocular lenses, or implants, restore good visual acuity with minimal magnification, nearly normal peripheral vision, fast rehabilitation, and no need for manipulation by the patient (Figure 9-3). An eye with a lens implant is referred to as *pseudophakic*. Even with an implant, glasses are needed to fine-tune distance vision and to provide clear near vision.

Contact lenses provide good restoration of aphakic vision, but they require dexterity, fastidious cleansing, and frequent replacement. Aphakic eyeglasses (cataract glasses) are used when implants or contact lenses cannot be used.

Figure 9-3 Intraocular lenses and cataract. This lens implant is being inserted into the eye after cataract removal. (Courtesy W.K. Kellogg Eye Center, University of Michigan.)

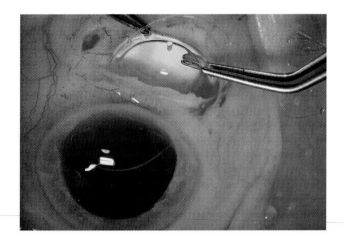

Unfortunately, they are heavy, unattractive, cause image magnification of 25% to 30% with distorted spatial perception, and require a long acclimation period.

Visual acuity is restored to precataract levels in more than 95% of uncomplicated cases. Rare complications include retinal detachment, macular edema, chronic uveitis, and keratopathy. However, nearly half of the patients who undergo extracapsular cataract surgery develop opacification of the posterior lens capsule within 6 months to 5 years postoperatively. Called a *secondary cataract* or an *aftercataract,* this opacification is treated by making a window in the capsule by means of the neodymium:yttrium-aluminum-garnet (Nd:YAG) laser. This laser capsulotomy, performed as a brief office procedure, has a generally favorable outcome.

Diabetic Retinopathy

AT A GLANCE

☐ Diabetic retinopathy is a vasculopathy that often causes visual loss resulting from macular edema and fibrovascular proliferation.

☐ Tight control of blood sugar markedly reduces the chances of developing retinopathy.

☐ Laser photocoagulation surgery can reduce by 50% the likelihood of severe visual loss but is most effective if performed before visual loss has occurred.

☐ Vitrectomy may restore some vision in patients whose disease is too advanced for photocoagulation.

☐ Because visual loss is often a late symptom and because of the difficulty of recognizing the early signs of diabetic retinopathy, physicians should counsel diabetic patients to maintain ophthalmologic care according to a recommended schedule.

Diabetic retinopathy is the retinal vascular disorder associated with diabetes mellitus. The pathologic progression involves vessel leakage, occlusion, fibrovascular proliferation, bleeding, and retinal detachment. Its pathogenesis is unclear.

Prevalence and Clinical Significance

Diabetic retinopathy is the leading cause of blindness among working-age Americans. Early diagnosis allows timely laser surgery, which significantly reduces visual loss.

Diagnosis

Diabetic retinopathy begins with a stage called *nonproliferative retinopathy.* Ophthalmoscopic findings, which reflect mural outpouching and leakage of incompetent capillaries, include microaneurysms, hard exudates, intraretinal hemorrhages, and macular edema. Microaneurysms, the earliest visible manifestations of diabetic retinopathy, are small red dots scattered in the posterior pole. Sometimes they are surrounded by a ring of lipid, or hard, exudate. Nonproliferative changes are asymptomatic unless the leakage and exudates involve the macula, the small area of the retina responsible for sharp central vision.

With increased duration of diabetes, further nonproliferative changes occur because of increased retinal ischemia. Among these changes, the most easily recognized are cotton-wool spots, discrete white areas with feathery edges. They reflect infarction of the nerve fiber layer of the retina.

The next stage, called *proliferative retinopathy,* includes retinal neovascularization and fibrous proliferation. Delicate new vessels form anterior to the retina and resemble a tangle of hair or a fish net lying just above the retinal surface or extending toward the vitreous cavity (Figure 9-4A). The new vessels may originate from the optic nerve head or from elsewhere on the retina.

Figure 9-4 Diabetic retinopathy. (**A**) Neovascularization on the retinal surface is due to chronic ischemia. (**B**) Panretinal photocoagulation has caused regression of neovascularization.

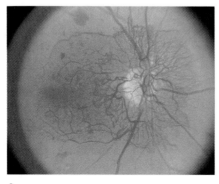

A

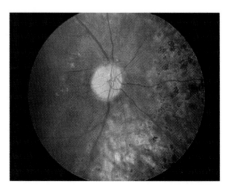

B

As these new vessels bleed into the retina or vitreous cavity, they stimulate proliferation of the fibrous scaffold that supports them. This scaffold eventually contracts and tugs on the retina, causing it to split or detach.

Many of the retinal changes of diabetes are difficult to identify through an undilated pupil. For this reason, it is advisable for physicians to refer diabetic patients for ophthalmologic evaluation according to a schedule based on age at diagnosis (see the Close-Up "Initial Ophthalmologic Examination of Diabetic Patients" in Chapter 2). Close collaboration between physicians and ophthalmologists in regular surveillance of these patients ensures optimal care.

Management

Tight control of blood sugar markedly reduces the chances of developing retinopathy.

National collaborative studies have shown that laser photocoagulation surgery can reduce by about 50% the likelihood of severe visual loss from both macular edema and proliferative retinopathy (Figure 9-4B). A critical finding of all studies is that photocoagulation is most effective if it is performed before patients experience visual loss.

Photocoagulation is not helpful in diabetic patients who have persistent vitreous hemorrhages or traction retinal detachments. For such patients, vitrectomy (removal of the vitreous body) is an option. About 60% to 80% of patients achieve improved vision following this procedure.

Glaucoma

AT A GLANCE

☐ Glaucoma, a major cause of blindness, consists of characteristic optic disc excavation and visual field defects. Elevated intraocular pressure is a common but not necessary feature.

☐ As a screening method for primary open-angle glaucoma, tonometry alone is inadequate. Detecting pathologic optic disc excavation by ophthalmoscopy is more effective. Physicians should refer for periodic ophthalmologic examination the high-risk patients—those over age 65, African-Americans, diabetic patients, and those with myopia or a family history of glaucoma.

☐ Treatment of glaucoma consists of medications and surgery aimed at lowering intraocular pressure.

The term *glaucoma* is applied to a number of conditions causing optic nerve damage, often in association with elevated intraocular pressure (IOP). The four main forms of glaucoma are primary open-angle, congenital, secondary, and angle-closure.

□ *Primary open-angle glaucoma,* making up more than 70% of all glaucoma cases, is a familial disease caused by acquired impairment of aqueous drainage through the trabecular meshwork. It is marked by progressive constriction of the field of vision, excavation of the optic nerve head, and often (but not always) elevated intraocular pressure.

□ *Congenital glaucoma,* a relatively rare form, is caused by a congenitally imperfect aqueous humor drainage mechanism.

□ *Secondary glaucoma* is the result of damage to the drainage mechanism by other intraocular diseases.

□ *Angle-closure glaucoma,* also a rare form, occurs when the root of the iris blocks the drainage mechanism in patients with anatomically shallow anterior chambers.

Prevalence and Clinical Significance

Primary open-angle glaucoma constitutes a major public health problem because it is common and patients are asymptomatic until vision is seriously compromised. Population-based surveys in the United States have yielded an estimated prevalence of about 1% among persons over age 40, rising to over 3% among those over 70. An estimated 16.2 persons per 100,000—possibly as many as 80,000 people—are legally blind from glaucoma in the United States. Although glaucomatous visual loss is irreversible, much of it may be preventable by early detection and treatment designed to lower intraocular pressure.

Congenital glaucoma is rare, but its diagnosis is urgent because timely surgery prevents permanent visual loss.

Secondary glaucoma is one of the most serious consequences of intraocular disease. It may also be an early or remote manifestation of ocular trauma that damages the drainage system.

Angle-closure glaucoma may strike suddenly, with very high intraocular pressure that must be relieved promptly to prevent permanent visual loss. There is also an indolent form of angle-closure glaucoma that, like primary open-angle glaucoma, is asymptomatic.

Diagnosis

Primary open-angle glaucoma is diagnosed by the presence of characteristic visual field loss and pathologic excavation (cupping) of the optic nerve head (Figure 9-5).

The most cost-effective method of screening for this form of glaucoma is debatable. In the past, physicians were urged to perform tonometry (measurement of IOP) and to refer any patient with IOP above 21 mm Hg to an ophthalmologist. Population-based studies have disclosed, however, that as many as 50% of patients with glaucoma have IOP levels below 21 mm Hg based on a single measurement. Lowering the cutoff level a few points fails to capture patients

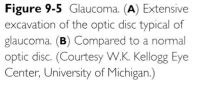

Figure 9-5 Glaucoma. (**A**) Extensive excavation of the optic disc typical of glaucoma. (**B**) Compared to a normal optic disc. (Courtesy W.K. Kellogg Eye Center, University of Michigan.)

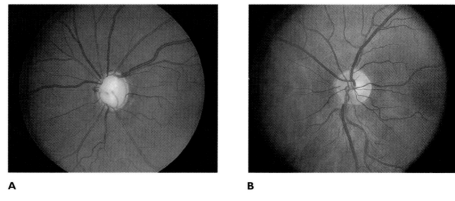

A   **B**

with normal-tension glaucoma. Moreover, about 85% of patients with IOP accurately measured above 21 mm Hg do not have glaucoma and will not develop it within 5 years. Studies also show that unless tonometry is performed frequently and with precise instruments, it is often inaccurate. For these reasons, the screening value of tonometry has been challenged.

The characteristic signs of primary open-angle glaucoma—optic nerve head excavation and visual field loss—are difficult to appreciate without the aid of specialized techniques. Recognizing subtotal cupping of the optic disc may require a fully dilated pupil and stereoscopic viewing devices. Glaucomatous visual field loss cannot be detected by confrontation visual field testing until it is far advanced.

Therefore, the detection of glaucoma may be more appropriately based on periodic ophthalmologic examination of individuals known to be at high risk by physicians or other community health care providers. The high-risk glaucoma groups are people over age 65, African-Americans, and individuals who have diabetes, myopia, or a family history of glaucoma.

Congenital glaucoma presents in a baby as tearing, photophobia, an enlarged eye, and a hazy cornea (Figure 9-6). Because the sclera of an infant is distensible, the high IOP enlarges the globe. The elevated IOP damages the corneal endothelium (causing corneal edema, tearing, and photophobia) and the optic nerve head (causing glaucomatous excavation and leading to vision loss). Infants

Figure 9-6 Congenital glaucoma. The infant's enlarged eyes and hazy corneas are caused by a malformed trabecular meshwork.

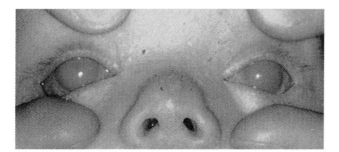

may show signs of congenital glaucoma within days of birth, although some cases develop later in the first year of life.

Secondary glaucoma is diagnosed when elevated IOP is found in patients with other ocular diseases (uveitis, diabetic retinopathy) or a history of severe ocular trauma. Magnified (slit-lamp) examination is necessary to detect the characteristic intraocular signs.

Angle-closure glaucoma may present acutely with severe ocular pain and blurred vision, a red eye, a hazy cornea, and markedly elevated IOP. The differential diagnosis includes other causes of an acute red eye.

Management

The treatment of all forms of glaucoma involves lowering IOP.

In *primary open-angle glaucoma,* medications are prescribed initially—many of which have substantial systemic side effects. If medications fail, laser surgery of the drainage channels may be effective. If not, a fistula is fashioned surgically between the anterior chamber and the subconjunctival space (Figure 9-7).

Figure 9-7 Primary open-angle glaucoma. (**A**) Normal flow of aqueous. (**B**) Impaired outflow through the trabecular meshwork. (**C**) Filtering surgery provides bypass for aqueous.

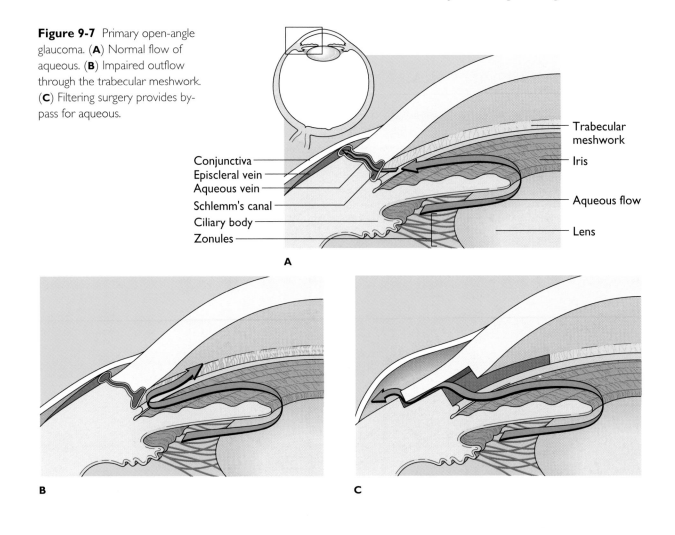

Trabecular meshwork

Conjunctiva
Episcleral vein
Aqueous vein
Schlemm's canal
Ciliary body
Zonules

Iris

Aqueous flow

Lens

A

B

C

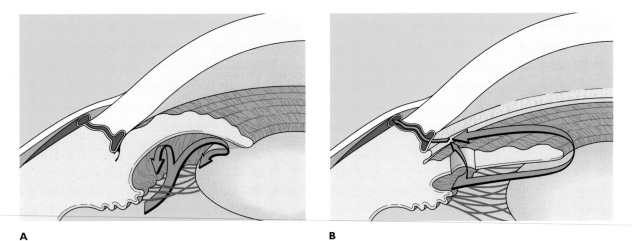

Figure 9-8 Acute angle-closure glaucoma. (**A**) The iris root occludes the trabecular meshwork. (**B**) Iridectomy restores access of aqueous to the trabecular meshwork.

The treatment of *congenital glaucoma* involves surgical separation (goniotomy) of the anterior chamber angle structures. If this operation fails, fistulizing procedures similar to those performed for primary open-angle glaucoma may be performed.

Treatment of *secondary glaucoma* consists of reducing inflammation as well as the measures used in primary open-angle glaucoma.

Treatment of *angle-closure glaucoma* involves emergent lowering of intraocular pressure with medications, followed by iridectomy performed with the laser or with incisional surgery (Figure 9-8).

Glaucomatous visual loss cannot be restored. But if the intraocular pressure is lowered substantially, progressive visual field loss may be prevented in a majority of cases.

Metastatic Cancers

AT A GLANCE

☐ Breast and lung carcinomas, leukemia, and lymphoma make up most metastases to the eye.

☐ Symptoms and signs include visual loss and choroidal masses.

☐ X-irradiation is the treatment of choice.

The eye may be the repository of metastatic carcinoma, principally from the breast and lung, but also as the result of leukemia or lymphoma.

Prevalence and Clinical Significance

Autopsy studies suggest that in patients who died from metastatic cancer, the eye was involved in 5% to 10% of cases. The ocular lesion may be the presenting sign in lung cancer and in immunoblastic lymphoma (primary central nervous system lymphoma). In leukemia, it may be the first clue to a relapse.

Diagnosis

Carcinoma metastatic to the eye most frequently involves the choroid, probably because of its high blood flow, but any structure within the eye (or orbit) may be affected. The patient typically complains of visual loss, and ophthalmoscopy discloses multiple yellow-gray, pancake-like choroidal masses with overlying retinal fluid. The differential diagnosis includes choroidal melanoma and non-neoplastic conditions.

Management

The treatment of all metastatic cancers to the eye is approximately 3000 cGy x-irradiation. Regression of signs usually occurs within days to weeks.

Optic Nerve Infarction in Giant-Cell Arteritis

AT A GLANCE

☐ Giant-cell arteritis, also known as *temporal* or *cranial arteritis,* may cause optic nerve infarction and permanent visual loss in up to 50% of patients.

☐ Once optic nerve infarction, also called *ischemic optic neuropathy,* has occurred in one eye, the chance is 1 in 3 that the other optic nerve will be infarcted within days unless high-dose corticosteroid treatment is instituted promptly.

Giant-cell (cranial, temporal) arteritis is an idiopathic inflammatory disease of medium-sized arteries that may cause infarction of the optic nerve.

Prevalence and Clinical Significance

Confined to older adults, giant-cell arteritis has a prevalence of 11 per 100,000 in those aged 50 or more and 27 per 100,000 in those aged 70 or more. Optic nerve infarction occurs in up to 50% of patients. Because high-dose corticosteroid treatment largely prevents this complication, early recognition of giant-cell arteritis is critical. Once infarction of one optic nerve has occurred, corticosteroids must be administered promptly to prevent infarction of the other optic nerve. Without treatment, the optic nerve in the other eye will be infarcted in one third of cases within days to weeks.

Diagnosis

The patient develops acute and painless loss of vision, usually in one eye. Visual loss may be minimal but is often devastating, even complete. A relative afferent pupillary defect is evident, and ophthalmoscopy discloses a swollen optic nerve head (Figure 9-9). These findings typically occur within weeks to months of the onset of a symptom complex made up of headache and jaw claudication (temporal arteritis syndrome), malaise, anorexia, fever, joint and muscle aches, and proximal weakness (polymyalgia rheumatic syndrome). The only laboratory sign is elevation of the sedimentation rate, but a normal sedimentation rate does not exclude the diagnosis. Pathologic confirmation may be obtained by finding granulomatous inflammation and fragmentation of the internal elastic membrane in a biopsy of the temporal artery.

Optic nerve infarction caused by giant-cell arteritis may occur in the absence of any systemic symptoms (occult arteritis). Sudden and persistent visual loss in an elderly adult who has a swollen optic nerve head must prompt consideration of this diagnosis. However, optic nerve infarction occurs far more commonly in patients who do not have giant-cell arteritis, but who have systemic hypertension, diabetes, or arteriosclerosis (nonarteritic optic nerve infarction).

Management

High-dose corticosteroids (oral prednisone 2 mg/kg/day or intravenous methylprednisolone 250 mg q6h) must be administered immediately. Doses are adjusted according to relief of the patient's systemic symptoms and normalization of the sedimentation rate. A temporal artery biopsy should be performed within a few days to confirm the diagnosis. Corticosteroids should generally not be administered for more than 1 year, as the disease typically will have run its course long before that time in most patients. Visual loss is irreversible.

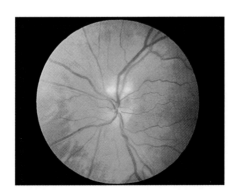

Figure 9-9 Optic nerve infarction (ischemic optic neuropathy) in giant-cell arteritis. Segmental pallid swelling of the optic disc is distinctive for infarction. (Courtesy W.K. Kellogg Eye Center, University of Michigan.)

Optic Neuritis

AT A GLANCE

☐   Optic neuritis is an autoimmune inflammation of the optic nerve that causes acute loss of vision, usually in one eye.

☐   Diagnosis depends on discovering subnormal visual function, a relative afferent pupillary defect, and no ophthalmoscopic signs of other causative conditions. Neuro-imaging and laboratory tests may be necessary to exclude a retrobulbar tumor or other inflammatory causes.

☐   Intravenous methylprednisolone, followed by oral prednisone, does not improve visual outcome, but significantly reduces new neurologic events in patients with abnormal MRI scans. Oral prednisone treatment by itself is not advocated because it provides no benefit and may predispose to more frequent recurrences of optic neuritis.

Optic neuritis is an autoimmune inflammation of the optic nerve that is either idiopathic or associated with multiple sclerosis. The principal target of the lymphocyte-mediated attack is the myelin sheath.

Prevalence and Clinical Significance

Although its exact prevalence is uncertain, optic neuritis is the most common optic neuropathy of early adulthood. Studies have shown that from 25% to 60% of individuals develop clinical multiple sclerosis within 15 years of the initial attack of optic neuritis.

Diagnosis

Patients with optic neuritis are typically between 18 and 45 years of age. They complain of acute monocular loss of vision and pain worsened by eye movement. Visual acuity or visual field is subnormal, and the affected eye almost always manifests a relative afferent pupillary defect. Findings on ophthalmoscopy are usually normal, although the optic nerve head may be swollen. There may be historical evidence of pre-existing multiple sclerosis or signs of multiple sclerosis on physical examination. If no evidence of multiple sclerosis exists, other inflammatory or compressive lesions of the optic nerve and chiasm must be considered. Evaluation may include blood tests and imaging studies.

Management

The Optic Neuritis Treatment Trial—a large, multicenter, randomized study—has shown that intravenous corticosteroid treatment does not improve final visual outcome, but significantly reduces the rate of new neurologic events in patients whose magnetic resonance imaging scans show abnormalities consistent with multiple sclerosis. Therefore, intravenous methylprednisolone (1 g per day for 3 days), followed by oral prednisone (1 mg/kg per day for 11 days), is recommended for treatment of such patients. Oral prednisone prescribed without the preceding intravenous methylprednisolone is of no benefit and appears to predispose patients to more frequent recurrences of optic neuritis.

Refractive Disorders

AT A GLANCE

- *Myopia* and *hyperopia* result from a mismatch between the eye's optical elements and its front-to-back length; *astigmatism* results from abnormal corneal curvature; *presbyopia* is a decline in accommodative power due to aging.

- In myopia, the eye's refracting power is excessive, so that distant objects are always out of focus unless the individual squints. High myopia is associated with a greater-than-average incidence of retinal detachment.

- In hyperopia, the eye's refracting power is inadequate, so that accommodation must be used to compensate. Refractive correction is generally not necessary until adulthood, when accommodation can no longer overcome the deficit.

- In astigmatism, the abnormal corneal curvature causes objects to be out of focus at all viewing distances.

Refractive disorders occur when the optical elements of the eye do not focus an image clearly on the retina (Figure 9-10). Myopia (nearsightedness), hyperopia (farsightedness), and astigmatism (distorted vision) are caused by an imbalance between the shape of the cornea and the anteroposterior diameter of the eye. All three may occur naturally as inherited disorders or as the result of ocular disease. Presbyopia is a refractive disorder resulting from the natural aging process. By middle age, the crystalline lens can no longer change its shape (accommodate) enough to provide a clear image of a near object. Over the ensuing two decades, the lens gradually loses all focusing ability.

Prevalence and Clinical Significance

Myopia accounts for more than 80% of all naturally occurring refractive disorders. The eye's refractive elements are relatively powerful, so that near objects are in focus but distant objects are not. The only way to see distant objects clearly without optical correction is to bypass the refractive apparatus by squinting (the Greek word *myein* means "to shut"). Thus, myopia may go undetected if visual acuity testing is performed at less than a 20-foot distance or the patient is allowed to squint.

Figure 9-10 Refractive disorders and their correction. (**A**) In emmetropia, or lack of refractive error, the light rays emanating from an object viewed at optical infinity come to focus on the retina without the need for refractive correction. (**B**) Uncorrected myopia: the eye's excessive refractive power causes light rays to focus in front of the retina. (**C**) Corrected myopia: a concave spherical lens counteracts the eye's excessive refractive power so that light rays now focus on the retina. (**D**) Uncorrected hyperopia: the eye's insufficient refractive power causes light rays to focus (theoretically) behind the retina. (**E**) Corrected hyperopia: a convex spherical lens supplements the eye's insufficient refractive power so that light rays now focus on the retina. (**F**) Uncorrected astigmatism: the eye's abnormal corneal curvature prevents a point focus of light. (**G**) Corrected astigmatism: a cylindrical lens causes light rays to focus on the retina.

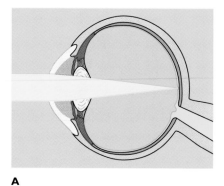

A

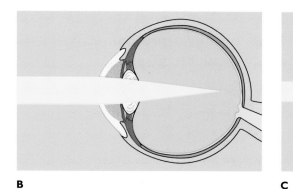

B

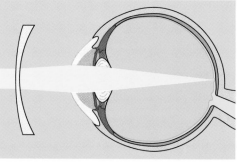

C

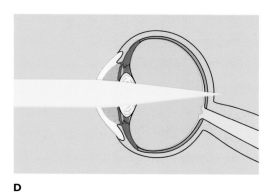

D

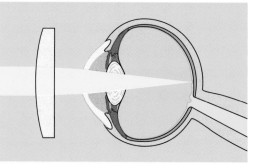

E

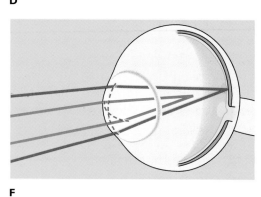

F

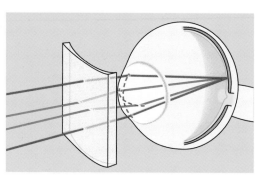

G

Myopia usually begins in the first decade of life, progresses at a variable rate, and typically stabilizes by the end of the second decade. Moderate-to-high myopia (greater than 5 diopters) is associated with a predisposition to retinal detachment. Patients should therefore have periodic ophthalmologic evaluation that includes indirect ophthalmoscopy.

Hyperopia makes up about 10% of naturally occurring refractive disorders. It is generally present at birth and tends to be nonprogressive. Children and young adults with hyperopia can usually achieve normal visual acuity by accommodating. However, as a result of constant accommodative effort, some hyperopic children develop inturning of the eyes (esotropia). Eyeglasses that correct the hyperopia may eliminate this esotropia (see "Strabismus" in this chapter).

Astigmatism constitutes about 40% of refractive disorders, occurring often in conjunction with myopia or hyperopia. Caused by irregular curvature of the cornea, it usually has its onset within the first decade and tends to progress little. Unlike myopia and hyperopia, which require spherical refractive correction, astigmatism requires cylindrical correction. Patients with more than 2 diopters of astigmatism may not be able to achieve clear vision with soft contact lenses.

Presbyopia affects everyone sooner or later, but most individuals become aware of it in their mid-40s, when their failing accommodative power no longer allows clear vision at normal reading distance.

Diagnosis

Patients who have myopia and astigmatism usually complain of unclear distance vision. But if the onset is slow or restricted to one eye, they may not be aware of their imperfect vision. Children typically tolerate quite poor vision before complaining. Hyperopic patients may not complain until adulthood, when accommodation can no longer compensate. They will then report eye ache or unclear vision when viewing near objects.

Presbyopia becomes apparent in middle age, when patients find near visual tasks, such as reading fine print, increasingly difficult. By contrast, patients who have been wearing a presbyopic correction for many years may discover that they can read more clearly *without* their correction—a phenomenon called *second sight*. Second sight derives from an increase in the index of refraction of the crystalline lens called *nuclear sclerosis,* which precedes cataract formation. The sclerosis causes progressive myopia, so that near objects become clear without optical aids. Unfortunately, this phenomenon causes distant objects to become blurred, requiring a myopic correction.

Management

Refractive disorders are corrected by eyeglasses, contact lenses, or corneal reshaping procedures. The choice depends on the nature of the refractive disor-

CLOSE-UP

CONTACT LENSES

☐ Contact lenses are worn by 25 million Americans: soft lenses (80%), rigid gas-permeable lenses (15%), and hard lenses (5%).

☐ Rigid gas-permeable lenses are most suitable for patients who cannot be fitted with soft contact lenses.

☐ Hard contact lenses have no advantages over rigid gas-permeable lenses and are being gradually discontinued.

☐ Soft lenses have the advantages of being comfortable, difficult to dislodge (as in sports), interchangeable with eyeglasses (without resulting in blurred vision), a rare cause of overwear symptoms, and available in disposable form.

☐ Soft lenses have the disadvantages of causing fluctuating vision, not correcting astigmatism above 2 diopters, requiring scrupulous hygiene, and accumulating surface deposits that may cause ocular irritation or injury.

☐ Extended-wear (overnight) soft contact lenses are convenient but, if worn for more than 7 days, may cause corneal ulcers that could permanently reduce vision. In 1989, the US Food and Drug Administration recommended a 7-day limit to wearing time. The figure shows a corneal ulcer due to *Pseudomonas aeruginosa* infection after the patient wore lenses for more than 7 days without removal, proper cleaning, and storage.

☐ Corneal infection is a risk even for daily-wear soft contact lens users if strict hygiene is not followed. The six rules are as follows:

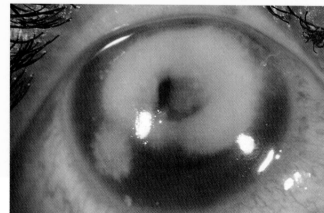

1. Wash hands before removing lens.
2. Use daily cleaner to remove deposits of fat.
3. Use weekly enzyme to remove protein deposits.
4. Use chemical or heat disinfection.
5. Use fresh commercial lens care solutions.
6. Clean and replace the lens case regularly.

Courtesy W. K. Kellogg Eye Center, University of Michigan.

der, the presence of other ocular abnormalities, patient comfort and desire, and cost. The Close-Up "Contact Lenses" provides information about this method of correcting refractive errors.

Neither eyeglasses nor contact lenses eliminate the optical mismatch that produces the refractive disorder; they merely compensate for it. Corneal reshaping procedures, on the other hand, do eliminate the mismatch by altering the refractive power of the cornea, the most important refractive element of the eye.

Among many reshaping procedures, the one called *radial keratotomy* has been the most successful. This surgical procedure involves a series of radial incisions of the cornea that weaken its focusing power. A national collaborative study has shown that it is capable of markedly—but not reliably—reducing moderate amounts (2 to 4 diopters) of myopia without serious visual risks. Another procedure, called *photorefractive keratectomy*, uses a laser to produce the same effect as radial keratotomy without the need for incisions. Its utility remains to be verified by large-scale studies.

Presbyopia is corrected by a lens that helps to focus near objects. In eyeglasses, alternatives are single-vision reading glasses, bifocals, trifocals, or multifocals (progressive-addition lenses). Bifocals offer clear vision for far distance and reading distance; trifocals offer clear vision for far distance, reading distance, and middle distance—kitchen counter, music stand, computer, drafting board. Multifocals, or "no-line" lenses, are a popular but expensive means of obtaining clear vision at far distance and for a continuous range that extends from middle to reading distance. Multifocals cause distortion of off-center images, a feature that some users cannot tolerate. Many patients who have moderate-to-high myopia prefer to remove their glasses and read without any optical correction.

In the correction of presbyopia with contact lenses, alternatives include monovision, in which one eye is corrected for distance vision and the other for near vision, and bifocal contact lenses, which have not yet been perfected.

Retinal Detachment

AT A GLANCE

☐ Retinal detachment is a separation of the sensory portion of the retina from its pigment epithelium.

☐ The initial event is often detachment of the vitreous from the retina, marked by the sensation of flashes of light and a shower of floaters. The patient should be immediately referred to an ophthalmologist to rule out a retinal hole. Sealing the hole usually prevents a retinal detachment.

☐ Once the retina has detached, the treatment is surgical. In retinal reattachment surgery, the prognosis for retaining 20/50 or better visual acuity falls from 85% to below 50% if the detachment has spread to involve the macula. Therefore, referral of a suspected detachment is especially emergent if visual acuity is still normal.

A retinal detachment is a separation of the neurosensory retina from its underlying pigment epithelial layer. Deprived of contact with the pigment epithelium, the rods and cones are unable to process visual information.

Most retinal detachments begin with detachment of the vitreous from the retina. The effects of aging, inflammation, or trauma on the overlying vitreous body lead to shrinkage and increased traction at its points of attachment to the retina, mostly in the retinal periphery. As the vitreous tugs on the retina, the patient hallucinates brief flashing lights (photopsias, phosphenes, Moore's lightning flashes). If the vitreous detaches itself from the retina, fibrous aggregates on its posterior surface will block light rays as they head toward the retina. This causes the appearance of "floaters" in the field of vision. If vitreous detachment occurs at a point where there is a retinal vessel, the vessel may rip open and discharge blood into the vitreous cavity, causing blurred vision. When the vitreous detaches forcefully at a point of strong adherence to the retina, a full-thickness retinal hole may result. Liquid portions of vitreous may then seep under the tear and detach the retina from the underlying pigment epithelium. As the retina detaches, the patient loses the field of vision corresponding to the detached region.

Risk factors for the development of a retinal detachment are aging, myopia, eye surgery, inflammation, trauma, a prior retinal detachment in the other eye, and a family history of retinal detachment.

Prevalence and Clinical Significance

Retinal detachments affect about 1 in 15,000 persons each year, most of them over age 50. If not treated promptly, the detachment may spread to involve the macula and compromise visual acuity. At that point, the prognosis for restoration of good vision worsens dramatically. Therefore, *a retinal detachment is always an ophthalmic emergency, and, paradoxically, even more of an emergency if visual acuity is still normal.*

A retinal detachment can be prevented by repairing the retinal hole before the vitreous seeps under it. Cryotherapy or laser surgery may be used to seal the hole in a relatively straightforward office procedure. Thus, any patient with a recent onset of floaters and flashes of light should be referred promptly to an ophthalmologist.

Diagnosis

The diagnosis of a retinal detachment is suggested by the triad of new flashes, floaters, and a visual field defect, but patients rarely report all three symptoms. Ultimately, the diagnosis rests on skilled ophthalmoscopy, including the use of an indirect ophthalmoscope, which allows a view of the retinal periphery, where most detachments originate (Figure 9-11).

Management

Treatment of retinal detachment is surgical. The surgeon locates the retinal hole (or holes), applies diathermy or cryotherapy to the area, and drains the fluid elevating the retina. The surgeon then sutures a constricting plastic band onto the sclera to shorten the diameter of the globe and relieve vitreous traction. Complex detachments may also require removal of the vitreous, internal photo-

Figure 9-11 Retinal detachment. The billowing gray folds of retina inferior to the optic disc signify detachment. (Courtesy W.K. Kellogg Eye Center, University of Michigan.)

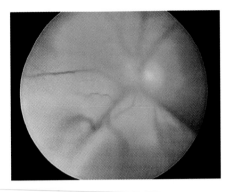

coagulation, and stripping of retinal membranes. After detachment surgery, patients experience moderate discomfort for about 3 days. A 2-day hospital stay is typical.

The prognosis for visual recovery depends on how long the detachment has been present and whether the macula is detached. If the macula is still attached at the time of surgery, 85% of patients will retain 20/50 acuity or better. If the macula is detached, less than 50% of patients will retain that degree of vision.

Retinal Vascular Occlusion

AT A GLANCE

☐ Retinal artery and vein occlusions usually result from thrombosis (artery and vein) or embolism (artery only). Amaurosis fugax (transient monocular blindness) is presumed to result from cardiac or carotid artery embolism. Systemic arteriosclerosis is the common underlying condition.

☐ The ophthalmoscopic manifestations of retinal arterial occlusion depend on the size of the occluded vessel. Cotton-wool spots and flame-shaped hemorrhages signify a small arteriolar blockage; retinal turbidity and a foveal cherry-red spot signify a large arteriolar blockage.

☐ The ophthalmoscopic appearance of a retinal vein occlusion consists primarily of blotchy surface hemorrhages. With substantial ischemia, cotton-wool spots are also seen.

☐ Treatment of acute central retinal arterial occlusion consists of reducing the intraocular pressure. Treatment of retinal vein occlusion consists of observing the patient carefully in ensuing months for the development of iris or retinal neovascularization, which may sometimes be reversed with retinal photocoagulation surgery.

Retinal vascular occlusions may involve either the arterial or the venous circulation. Retinal arterial occlusions most often result from embolism or thrombosis;

venous occlusions result from thrombosis. Transient monocular visual loss (amaurosis fugax) is presumed to result from retinal emboli that originate in the cervical carotid artery or the heart, temporarily plugging the arterial vascular tree, breaking up, and moving down the bloodstream. Because ischemia has been brief, visual function recovers.

Prevalence and Clinical Significance

Retinal vascular occlusions, both arterial and venous, are usually a sign of systemic arteriosclerosis. Other considerations are cardiogenic emboli (arterial only), vasculitis, hypercoagulable states (arterial or venous), and increased orbital or retro-orbital pressure (venous only). Arterial occlusions produce irreversible deficits; venous occlusions often produce reversible deficits but carry a long-term risk of visual complications from ocular neovascularization.

Diagnosis

A small arteriolar occlusion produces a flame-shaped hemorrhage or a cotton-wool spot, a small white patch in the superficial retina that obscures the retinal vessels. The lesions are so small that patients typically do not notice any loss of vision.

A large arteriolar occlusion causes retinal turbidity, and the fovea appears cherry-red if the infarction involves that region (Figure 9-12A). The patient notices a sudden, painless loss of central or paracentral vision.

If the entire retinal arterial tree has been occluded (central retinal artery occlusion), the cause may be an in situ thrombus or an embolus. But if a large branch vessel has been blocked (branch retinal artery occlusion), the cause is an embolus. The diagnosis of retinal embolism is firmer if a yellowish-white plug

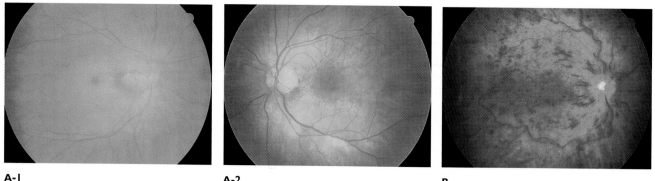

A-1   A-2   B

Figure 9-12 Retinal vascular occlusion. (**A-1**) In central retinal artery occlusion, portions of the retina are turbid (milky) and a cherry-red spot appears at the fovea. (**A-2**) Compare with the normal fellow eye. (**B**) In central retinal vein occlusion, hemorrhages cover the retinal surface and the veins are dilated. (Courtesy W.K. Kellogg Eye Center, University of Michigan.)

(Hollenhorst plaque) is seen in the retinal arteriole. One or more such plaques may also be discovered in patients who have reported transient monocular visual loss.

Central retinal vein occlusion (CRVO) causes acute, painless monocular visual loss, but not quite as quickly as does occlusion of the artery. Vision decreases over a period of hours. Ophthalmoscopic examination reveals a "blood-and-thunder optic fundus"—massive nerve fiber and preretinal hemorrhage (Figure 9-12B). If the venous stasis is severe enough, the arterial supply to the retina will be so slowed that infarction occurs (ischemic CRVO), marked by cotton-wool spots. As weeks go by, the blood is gradually absorbed, allowing substantial recovery of vision in the nonischemic CRVO cases. In some cases, the vein occlusion is limited to a branch (BRVO). The visual prognosis is better in BRVO than in CRVO.

Management

Treatment of a large retinal artery occlusion is of uncertain efficacy. Confronted with a patient whose visual loss from retinal artery occlusion is less than 8 hours old, most ophthalmologists try to lower the intraocular pressure vigorously (by ocular massage, anterior chamber aspiration of aqueous humor, intravenous acetazolamide, or oral glycerol) in hopes of breaking up the intravascular clot.

There is no immediate treatment for retinal vein occlusion. However, such patients need to be observed carefully, because a substantial number will develop neovascularization of the iris or retina, often within months of the occlusion. If the neovascularization involves the iris, it can lead to closure of the anterior chamber angle and intractable glaucoma. Neovascularization of the retina leads to macular edema, retinal bleeding, and retinal detachment, as in diabetic retinopathy. Usually, the new vessel growth can be rapidly reversed by retinal laser photocoagulation surgery.

The workup of transient monocular visual loss includes an evaluation of arteriosclerotic risk factors and noninvasive study of the heart or carotid artery for sources of emboli.

Retinoblastoma

AT A GLANCE

☐ Retinoblastoma is the most common primary intraocular malignancy of childhood.

☐ Leukocoria (cat's-eye reflex) or strabismus is the principal indicator leading to discovery of the condition.

☐ Screening children for red reflexes and strabismus promotes early detection; the smaller the tumor on diagnosis, the better the prognosis for survival and sight.

Retinoblastoma, the most common primary intraocular malignancy of childhood, is made up of primitive neuroblasts. The development of this tumor is ascribed to a defect in a retinoblastoma gene, which is believed to protect against malignancy.

Prevalence and Clinical Significance

Retinoblastoma affects 1 in every 18,000 live births. An estimated 250 to 500 new cases are diagnosed in the United States each year, mostly before age 3. Only 6% of cases have a family history of retinoblastoma; in these families, the tumor is passed by autosomal dominant transmission with nearly total penetrance. Of the sporadic cases, 25% are genetically transmitted; binocular involvement with retinoblastoma is a sign that the tumor will be transmitted.

Untreated retinoblastoma causes death by brain and visceral metastasis in nearly all cases. The smaller the tumor at diagnosis, the better the prognosis for survival and for sight in the affected eye.

Diagnosis

Retinoblastoma is usually discovered when a young child is found to have leukocoria (cat's-eye reflex) or strabismus (Figure 9-13). Thus, it is important to screen infants and young children for red fundus reflexes and strabismus (see "Strabismus" in this chapter). Ophthalmoscopic examination will reveal one or more white masses growing from the retina. However, several nonneoplastic exudative and dysplastic lesions of the retina may be mistaken for retinoblastoma. A helpful indicator of retinoblastoma is calcification, demonstrated on CT imaging scans.

Management

Removal of the eye (enucleation) has been the traditional treatment for advanced retinoblastoma in one eye. The second eye is treated with external or

Figure 9-13 Leukocoria (cat's-eye reflex) in retinoblastoma. The tumor behind the pupil turns the red reflex to a white reflex.

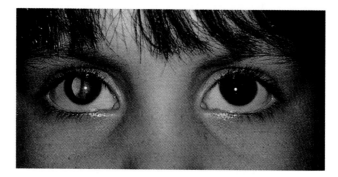

plaque radiotherapy; chemotherapy and cryotherapy are other options. Survival has reached 90% with these methods. The ability to preserve useful vision varies with the extent of the tumor at diagnosis, ranging from 32% to 95%.

Retinopathy of Prematurity

AT A GLANCE

☐ Retinopathy of prematurity (ROP) is a potentially blinding disease of infants of low gestational age.

☐ Cryotherapy performed at an intermediate stage of ROP reduces progression to the vision-threatening stages of the disease.

☐ Followup ophthalmoscopy is indicated for at-risk infants whose last examination in the nursery was negative for ROP but whose retinal vasculature was not mature at the time of that examination.

Retinopathy of prematurity is a proliferation of peripheral retinal vessels in babies who have one or more of these risk factors: (1) birth weight of 1250 g or less, (2) gestational age of 32 weeks or less, (3) mechanical ventilation, and (4) requirement for oxygen supplementation. The term *retinopathy of prematurity* (ROP) replaces the name *retrolental fibroplasia* (RLF), which refers to the white mass of fibrous detached retina seen behind the lens of the eye in the late stages of this illness (Figure 9-14).

The pathogenesis of ROP remains uncertain. Exposed to the relatively oxygen-rich extrauterine environment, the immature retinal circulation of the low-birth-weight infant develops abnormal new blood vessels at the junction of the vascular and avascular regions of the retina. At its extreme, ROP leads to irreparable complete retinal detachment and blindness.

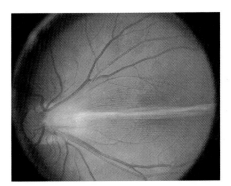

Figure 9-14 Retinopathy of prematurity. The horizontal preretinal yellow-white fibrous band reflects chronic ischemia and neovascularization in the peripheral retina. (Courtesy W.K. Kellogg Eye Center, University of Michigan.)

Although oxygen administration is no longer considered a major factor in the development of ROP, arterial oxygen levels in these premature infants should be carefully monitored and maintained at partial pressures below 100 mm Hg.

Prevalence and Clinical Significance

The most critical risk factor for ROP appears to be gestational age, but because estimates of gestational age may be inaccurate, birth weight is a substitute measure. ROP rarely occurs in neonates weighing more than 2000 g at birth. Its prevalence in the neonate weighing 1000 g to 1250 g is 20%, rising to 60% to 80% in the neonate weighing less than 1000 g.

A recent nationwide collaborative trial has disclosed that timely cryotherapy of the peripheral retina may save sight, emphasizing the need for early detection of infants with active ROP.

Diagnosis

Infants whose birth weight is 1250 g or less should be screened between 5 and 7 weeks after birth. Examination requires the use of indirect ophthalmoscopy after wide pupil dilation. Followup examination of infants is made on the basis of the clinical findings.

The description of the neonate's fundus is based on a classification for ROP. The active stages (1 to 5) are documented in specific regions of the eye. Each stage is determined by ophthalmoscopy, with stage 1 defined by the presence of a distinct line at the junction of the vascular and avascular retina. Stage 2 manifests an elevated ridge in this same region. Stage 3 adds the more ominous fibrovascular proliferation. Stage 4 has subtotal retinal detachment, and stage 5 has total retinal detachment. The term *plus disease* is a modifier applied to these stages that denotes dilation of retinal vessels and indicates aggressive disease.

Management

Cryotherapy is indicated once ophthalmoscopy discloses stage 3 plus disease involving more than 150° of the retina. The rationale for this treatment is to ablate the avascular retina, presumably destroying the factors that give rise to the new blood vessels—much as is done in diabetic retinopathy. Once stages 4 and 5 occur, in which the retina is detached in varying degrees, extensive reattachment surgery is advocated, but improvement in visual function has been discouragingly limited.

Even if babies show no signs of ROP while in the newborn nursery, they remain at risk for later development of the disease if the retina is not fully vascularized prior to discharge from the hospital. Therefore, after infants leave the nursery, followup care should be continued with an ophthalmologist until vascularization is complete.

Strabismus

AT A GLANCE

☐ Strabismus, or ocular misalignment, affects 4% of children, causing amblyopia, reduced stereopsis, and a deformed appearance.

☐ The four common childhood forms are visual deprivation, infantile esotropia, accommodative esotropia, and early childhood exotropia.

☐ Treatment includes correcting the underlying causes, eliminating the amblyopia, and realigning the eyes by operating on the extraocular muscles.

☐ Early detection and treatment produce a greater chance of permanent realignment without the development of amblyopia.

Strabismus is a misalignment of the two eyes, described according to the direction of misalignment. For example, esotropia refers to an inturning of the eye; exotropia, an outward turning of the eye; and hypertropia, an upturning of the eye.

The pathogenesis of childhood-onset strabismus is quite different from that acquired in adulthood, in which cranial-nerve palsies, ocular myopathies, and myasthenia gravis are predominant causes. In children, in whom the pathogenesis is frequently uncertain, the most common forms are described below.

☐ *Strabismus of visual deprivation* often develops when clear vision is interrupted in one or both eyes. The most serious underlying causes are retinoblastoma and optic nerve or chiasmal tumors. Strabismus may be the only outward sign of these tumors.

☐ *Infantile esotropia,* an idiopathic form of strabismus, is present at birth or develops in the first months of life. Although sometimes found in developmentally retarded children, it is more commonly an isolated condition.

☐ *Accommodative esotropia* occurs in children who have a hyperopic refractive error and must therefore accommodate to see clearly. As part of this extra accommodative effort, convergence is triggered and esotropia may develop. Accommodative esotropia usually first appears between 2 and 4 years of age, but may appear as early as age 2 months.

☐ *Childhood exotropia* usually first becomes evident between ages 3 and 6. A frequent early report is that the child's eye drifts outward in bright sunlight. Although no underlying cause is usually present, visual deprivation must always be ruled out.

Prevalence and Clinical Significance

Strabismus affects an estimated 4% of children. Although the alignment deformity may be the most noticeable feature, its most important consequences are amblyopia and reduced stereopsis. Early correction of strabismus largely prevents these consequences.

Figure 9-15 Strabismus. (**A**) Accommodative esotropia. (**B**) Eyeglasses align the eyes by eliminating the need for accommodation. (Courtesy W.K. Kellogg Eye Center, University of Michigan.)

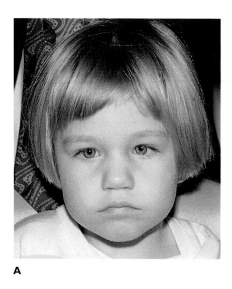

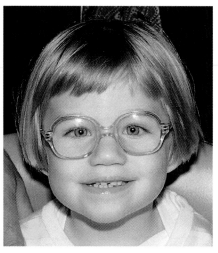

A

B

Diagnosis

The diagnosis of strabismus is made by means of the corneal light reflection and cover tests.

Management

The treatment of all forms of strabismus follows a three-step approach: (1) eliminate the underlying cause, (2) correct the amblyopia, and (3) attempt to restore normal ocular alignment with extraocular muscle surgery. For example, in managing the strabismus of visual deprivation secondary to retinoblastoma, the first step is to treat the tumor. In cases of accommodative esotropia, treatment starts with corrective lenses (Figure 9-15). In general, the sooner treatment is begun, the more likely the eyes will be properly realigned without developing amblyopia.

Uveal Melanoma

AT A GLANCE

☐ Melanomas in the iris, ciliary body, or choroid are the most common primary intraocular malignancies in adults.

☐ Iris melanomas and some ciliary body melanomas can be excised with preservation of vision and life. Choroidal melanomas are the most life-threatening and difficult to treat.

Uveal melanoma, the most common primary intraocular malignancy of adulthood, may arise in the iris, ciliary body, or choroid (Figure 9-16). No definite risk factors have been identified.

Prevalence and Clinical Significance

This malignancy has an incidence of 5 to 8 per million. It occurs most frequently in patients over age 40, with the incidence rising steeply after age 60. The larger the melanoma at diagnosis, the more likely it has already metastasized.

Diagnosis

Iris melanoma is discovered when a patient or physician notes a discoloration of the iris or a distortion of the pupil. Ciliary body and choroidal melanomas are found on routine ophthalmologic examination, when a patient complains of poor vision, or when a patient or physician notes a black lesion on the sclera.

Benign uveal masses, especially in the choroid, may simulate melanomas. Definitive diagnosis depends on a combination of ophthalmoscopy, ultrasound, and fluorescein angiography. Unfortunately, biopsy of the choroid is incompatible with preservation of vision.

Management

Iris melanomas are treated (by excision) only if they are growing. Generally of low-grade malignancy, they do not affect vision or life span. Ciliary body and choroidal melanomas, which are more malignant than iris melanomas, are usually treated (by excision or radiation). Vision may be preserved after excision of a ciliary body melanoma. The optimal treatment of a choroidal melanoma is controversial; a collaborative study currently under way is comparing the effects of enucleation, external-beam radiotherapy, and plaque radiotherapy on survival.

Figure 9-16 Ocular melanomas. (**A**) Iris melanoma. (**B**) Choroidal melanoma, a round, brownish lesion deep to the retina. (Courtesy W.K. Kellogg Eye Center, University of Michigan.)

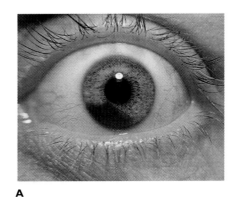

A

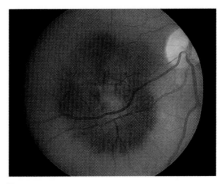

B

Common Questions From Patients

General Vision

Q: When should my child's eyes be examined by an ophthalmologist?

A: In the absence of specific concerns, children should have routine screening examinations at about age 6 months, 3 years, and 5 years. Specific concerns that require prompt evaluation include an absent red reflex, suspicions that the child is not seeing well, indications of a "lazy" or wandering eye, or hereditary factors that might predispose the child to eye disease (see Chapter 2).

Q: Is my child likely to inherit my need for glasses?

A: If both parents wear glasses, their offspring are likely to need them too. But when only one parent has a vision problem, it's impossible to predict.

Q: Will sitting too close to the television set hurt my child's eyes?

A: No, there is no scientific evidence that television emits rays that are harmful to the eyes.

Q: My child sits close to the television set and holds books extremely close to his eyes. Should I have his eyes checked?

A: Children have stronger focusing ability than adults and enjoy looking at things up close because they become more absorbed that way. However, if in addition to holding things close, the child is not seeing things clearly at normal viewing distances, he should be taken for an eye examination.

Q: Since I've become middle-aged, why have I been unable to read without glasses?

A: The ability to focus on near objects (accommodation) decreases steadily with age. Referred to as *presbyopia,* this condition becomes noticeable at around age 40, at which time glasses or bifocals are usually prescribed (see Chapter 9).

Q: Will working at a computer screen hurt my eyes?

A: There is no evidence that working at a computer damages the eyes. However, long hours of work with few interruptions can be fatiguing to the eyes, neck, back, and legs. These suggestions are often helpful: Take periodic breaks and look off in the distance, rather than reading or doing close work during the breaks. People who wear bifocals may adjust the work station for easier viewing through their reading lenses by lowering the monitor screen, angling it upward a few degrees, or raising the chair. Trifocals provide clearer vision for middle distance than do bifocals, especially for individuals over 50 years of age.

Q: Is my vision good enough for driving a car?

A: Most states require licensees to have a best-corrected vision of at least 20/40 in one eye for day and night driving, while those with vision corrected to no better than 20/70 in one eye are generally limited to daytime driving. In addition, some states require a minimum level of peripheral vision. For specific requirements, check with the state motor vehicle department.

Q: Do eye exercises improve vision?

A: No, but eye muscle exercises may be helpful in reducing double vision in convergence insufficiency, an uncommon condition in which the eyes go out of alignment when viewing a target at reading distance.

Q: Will reading in dim light hurt my eyes?

A: No, but most people find it more comfortable to read with proper lighting—lighting bright enough to provide good illumination but not so bright as to cause glare.

Q: Is it harmful to use my eyes too much?

A: No, the eyes are not subject to being "overused" or "used up."

Q: If one eye is damaged, does that put a strain on the other eye?

A: No, not in the sense of making it "work harder" or fatiguing more easily. However, people with vision in only one eye should take every precaution for eye safety to preserve vision in the remaining eye. (See the Close-Up "Prevention of Eye Injuries" in Chapter 5.)

Eyeglasses

Q: Why is it that after using bifocals for many years, now, at age 70, I can suddenly read without my glasses?

A: This myopic condition, called *second sight,* is caused by age-related changes in the lens and may be a forewarning of cataract formation. In conjunction with second sight, patients may also notice decreased visual acuity for distant objects. This can usually be overcome with a new distance correction.

Q: How often do glasses need to be changed?

A: Glasses need changing only when they no longer provide adequate correction, and not on any predetermined schedule. The frequency of change is generally related to age and status of eye health. In nearsighted teenagers or patients who have had cataract surgery, glasses may have to be changed several times a year. In young adults, prescriptions are generally more stable—in some cases for 10 years or more. In middle-aged adults with presbyopia, prescriptions typically need to be adjusted every 2 to 5 years until age 60, after which further changes are rare unless cataracts develop or eye surgery is performed.

Q: What type of material should I choose for my eyeglass lenses?

A: Several types of glass and plastic materials are available, each with different properties. Glass has some advantages: it is available in lenses that darken in bright sun (Photogray), and it is relatively scratch-proof. Plastic is lighter than glass, less likely to shatter on impact, but more likely to become scratched. Among the plastics available, polycarbonate plastic is the most shatter-proof and should be prescribed when safety is a consideration, particularly in patients with vision in only one eye. (See the Close-Up "Prevention of Eye Injuries" in Chapter 5.)

Q: Are sunglasses good for my eyes?

A: There are no adverse health consequences to wearing sunglasses during the day. In fact, sunglasses, especially those that wrap around and filter ultraviolet (UV) light, may protect against cataract formation. Clear lenses that filter UV light may offer greater protection than dark lenses, because the eyes are exposed to more light, resulting in greater pupillary constriction and, therefore, less light entering the eyes. It is hazardous to wear darkly tinted lenses when driving at night.

Contact Lenses

Q: Can my child wear contact lenses during sports activities?
A: Yes, contact lenses provide excellent vision for sports. However, they do not protect the eyes from injury. Therefore, when participating in sports, especially ball sports for which helmets are not generally worn (racquet sports, baseball, and

basketball), contact lens wearers should also use sports safety glasses with poly-carbonate lenses. (See the Close-Up "Prevention of Eye Injuries" in Chapter 5.)

Q: Can I use my eyeglass prescription to buy over-the-counter contact lenses?

A: No. In contrast to an eyeglass prescription, which provides only the refractive correction, a contact lens prescription contains specifications for fitting the lens on the eye, including lens diameter, base curve (shape), and thickness. Moreover, a new contact lens prescription must be carefully fitted by an eye care specialist to avoid serious adverse reactions.

Q: Can soft contact lenses correct for astigmatism?

A: This depends on the degree of astigmatism. Although some astigmatic patients can be fitted with special types of soft contact lenses, patients with more than 2 diopters of astigmatism probably need rigid gas-permeable lenses.

Q: Rather than a commercial saline solution, is it safe for me to clean my contact lenses with a homemade solution made from salt tablets?

A: No, contact lens wearers should use *only* commercial saline solutions. Recent studies have shown that homemade solutions put patients at risk for corneal infections from *Acanthamoeba*.

Q: In addition to my regularly scheduled visits, under what circumstances should I see my ophthalmologist to check my contact lenses?

A: A red eye, eye pain, or a noticeable change in vision should prompt a visit to an ophthalmologist.

Eye Diseases and Conditions

Q: I have a cataract, but my vision is good. Do I need surgery?

A: As long as patients are happy with their vision and it satisfies the demands of daily living (including licensing requirements for driving), surgery is usually unnecessary. However, surgery is sometimes indicated for medical reasons other than the cataract, such as for some forms of glaucoma and retinal disease. Patients should check with their ophthalmologist if they are concerned. (See "Cataract" in Chapter 9.)

Q: Can cataracts be removed with lasers?

A: No, cataract surgery involves cutting and other methods to remove most, but not all, of a patient's lens. However, patients are justifiably confused because the Nd:YAG (neodymium:yttrium-aluminum-garnet) laser is often used several weeks or months after such cataract surgery to clear an opening in the remaining, opacified lens capsule. The laser surgery is painless, quick, and performed in an outpatient setting. (See "Cataract" in Chapter 9.)

Q: What is a "lazy" eye, and how can I tell if my child has one?

A: A lazy eye is one that has reduced vision, usually arising from either strabismus (crossed eyes) or a large refractive error. Known as *amblyopia*, the condition is detected by the physician who measures visual acuity. In children under 3 years of age in whom visual acuity is difficult to assess, the physician may make a presumptive diagnosis of amblyopia based on whether the child has a wandering eye or objects to having one eye covered. (See "Amblyopia" in Chapter 9.)

Q: Is "pink eye" contagious?

A: Viral conjunctivitis, the most common form of pink eye, is extremely contagious (see Chapter 4). Patients should avoid touching their eyes and should wash their hands frequently, drying them with disposable towels. Ideally, they should also avoid communal activities for at least 5 days after the clinical onset of the disease. In contrast, bacterial conjunctivitis is a relatively rare cause of pink eye and is not particularly contagious.

Q: I have age-related macular degeneration. Should I be taking zinc tablets?

A: A few studies have suggested an association between macular degeneration and low levels of zinc in the blood. Accordingly, some ophthalmologists advise their patients with age-related macular degeneration to take 50 mg of zinc daily, 1 hour after a meal, to prevent further retinal damage. However, the scientific validity of zinc therapy for either restoring sight or preventing further visual loss remains to be demonstrated conclusively.

Eye Care Professionals

Q: What is the difference between an ophthalmologist, an optometrist, and an optician?

A: These three types of eye care professionals are described in the table below.

Title	Degree	Licensed to	Years of Training	Practice
Ophthalmologist	MD	Practice medicine and surgery	4 years of college, 4 years of medical school, 1 year of internship, 3 years of residency	Diagnoses and treats all eye diseases; performs eye surgery; prescribes and fits glasses and contact lenses
Optometrist	OD	Practice optometry	2 to 4 years of college, 4 years of optometric college	Determines the need for glasses and contact lenses and prescribes optical correction; screens for abnormalities of eye; treats visual disturbances with glasses and contact lenses
Optician		Dispense (make) optical aids	Varies from preceptorships to 2 years of opticianry school	Fits, adjusts, and dispenses glasses, contact lenses, and other optical devices on written prescription of a licensed physician (ophthalmologist) or optometrist

Illustrated Ophthalmic Anatomy

Figure B-1 External eye and lacrimal system

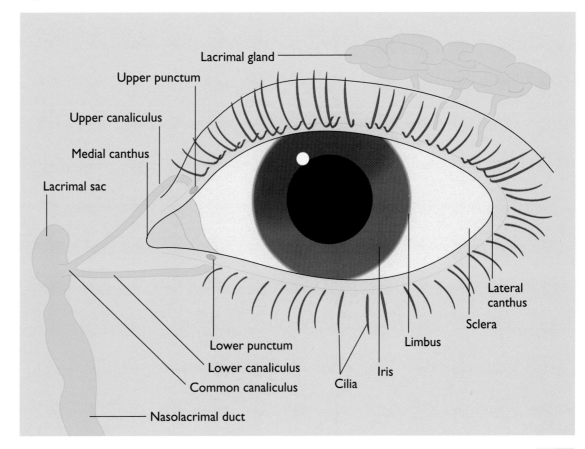

Figure B-2 Cross section of the eye

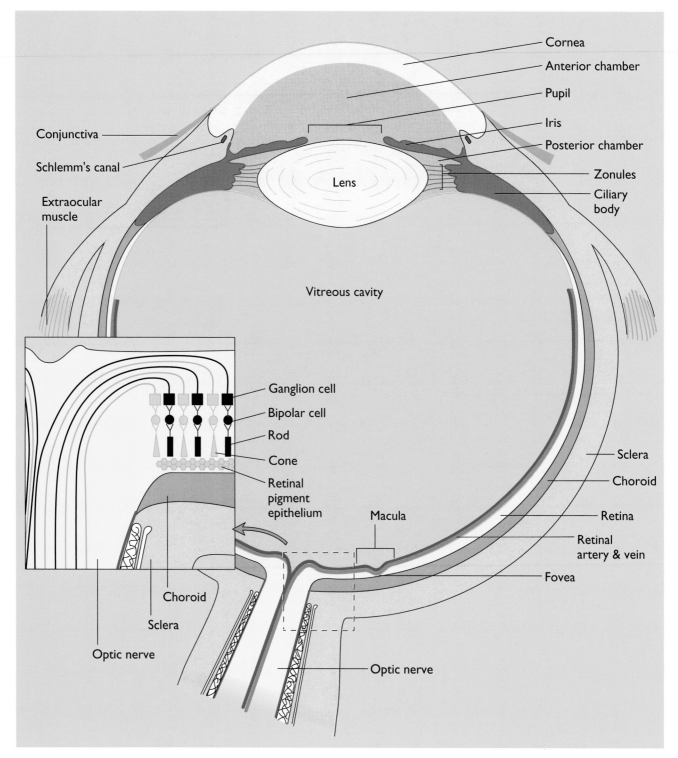

Figure B-3 Sagittal section of the eye in the orbit

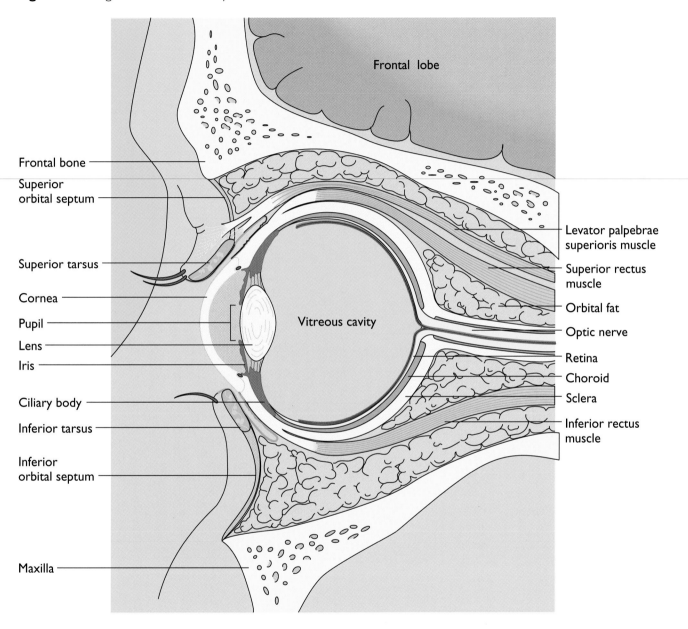

Frontal lobe

Frontal bone

Superior
orbital septum

Superior tarsus

Cornea

Pupil

Lens

Iris

Ciliary body

Inferior tarsus

Inferior
orbital septum

Maxilla

Vitreous cavity

Levator palpebrae
superioris muscle

Superior rectus
muscle

Orbital fat

Optic nerve

Retina

Choroid

Sclera

Inferior rectus
muscle

Figure B-4   Cross section of the eyelid

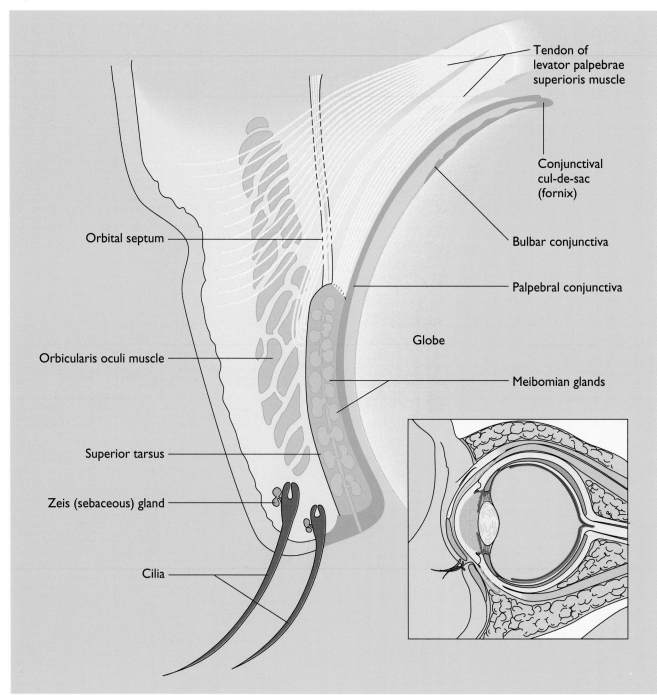

Tendon of levator palpebrae superioris muscle

Conjunctival cul-de-sac (fornix)

Bulbar conjunctiva

Palpebral conjunctiva

Globe

Meibomian glands

Orbital septum

Orbicularis oculi muscle

Superior tarsus

Zeis (sebaceous) gland

Cilia

Figure B-5   Normal fundus

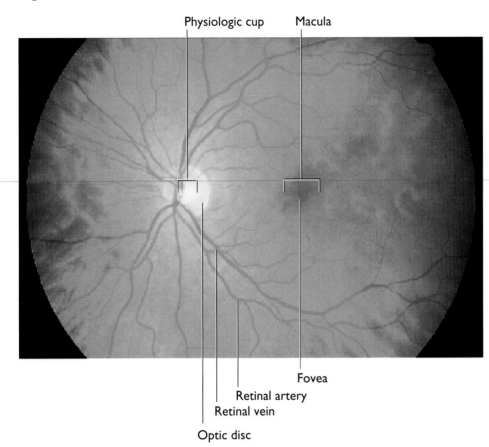

Physiologic cup   Macula

Fovea

Retinal artery

Retinal vein

Optic disc

Figure B-6   Visual pathway

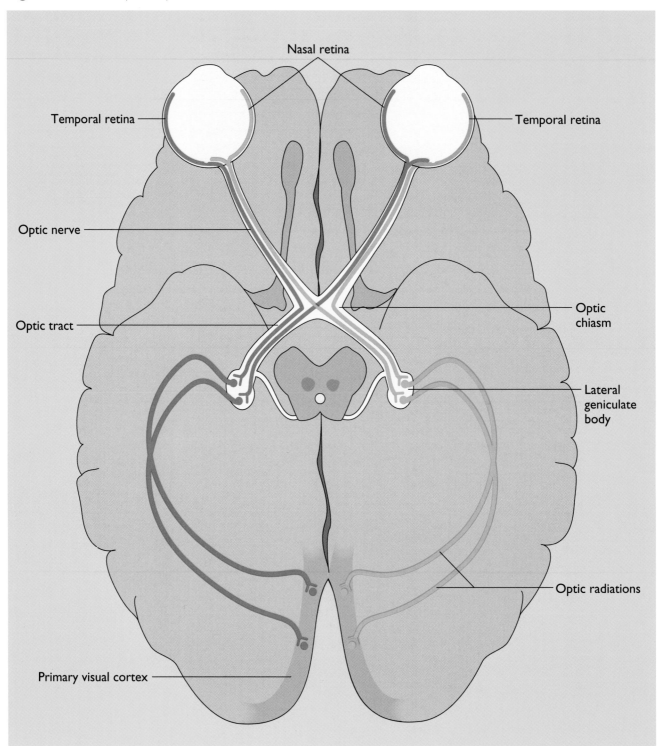

Annotated Resources

Introductory Textbooks

Goldberg S: *Ophthalmology Made Ridiculously Simple.* Miami: MedMaster; 1990. A light-hearted introduction to ophthalmology, emphasizing anatomy illustrated with cartoons; popular among medical students.

Kanski JJ: *Clinical Ophthalmology: A Systematic Approach.* London: Butterworths; 1989. A well-illustrated text, aimed primarily at ophthalmology residents.

Newell FW: *Ophthalmology: Principles and Concepts.* 7th ed. St Louis: Mosby–Year Book; 1992. A well-written standard hard-cover introduction to ophthalmology.

Vaughan DG, Asbury T, Riordan-Eva P: *General Ophthalmology.* 13th ed. Norwalk, CT: Appleton & Lange; 1992. A popular soft-cover comprehensive introduction to ophthalmology, aimed primarily at medical students and beginning ophthalmology residents.

Comprehensive Textbooks

Duke-Elder S: *System of Ophthalmology.* St Louis: CV Mosby Co; 1976. An excellent source for clinical descriptions but obviously out of date.

Tasman W, Jaeger EA, eds: *Duane's Clinical Ophthalmology.* Philadelphia: JB Lippincott Co. Six volumes revised annually; the most extensive general reference available.

Specialized Textbooks

Gold DH, Weingeist TA: *The Eye in Systemic Disease.* Philadelphia: JB Lippincott Co; 1990. Brief essays on ophthalmic manifestations of systemic diseases.

Hedges TR III: *Consultation in Ophthalmology.* Toronto: BC Decker; 1987. A concise soft-cover compendium of ophthalmic manifestations of systemic diseases.

Miller NR: *Walsh & Hoyt's Clinical Neuro-ophthalmology.* Baltimore: Williams & Wilkins; 1982-1990. A four-volume authoritative source emphasizing the neurologic and systemic aspects of ophthalmic diseases.

Nelson LB, Calhoun JH, Harley RD: *Pediatric Ophthalmology.* 3rd ed. Philadelphia: WB Saunders Co; 1991. The most comprehensive source for ophthalmic diseases of children.

General Manuals

Berson FG, ed: *Basic Ophthalmology for Medical Students and Primary Care Residents.* 6th ed. San Francisco: American Academy of Ophthalmology; 1993. Covers most of the topics presented in this book, but more briefly.

Pavan-Langston D: *Manual of Ocular Diagnosis and Therapy.* Boston: Little, Brown and Co; 1991. A spiral-bound "Washington manual–style" presentation.

Roy FH: *Ocular Differential Diagnosis.* 5th ed. Philadelphia: Lea & Febiger; 1993. Lists of differential diagnoses by symptoms.

Therapeutics and Toxicology Manuals

Fraunfelder FT, Roy FH, eds: *Current Ocular Therapy 3.* Philadelphia: WB Saunders Co; 1990. Essays on the treatment of ophthalmic diseases.

Grant WM: *Toxicology of the Eye.* 3rd ed. Springfield, IL: Charles C Thomas; 1986. A classic source for ophthalmic side effects of ocular and systemic medications.

Pavan-Langston D, Dunkel EC: *Handbook of Ocular Drug Therapy and Ocular Side Effects of Systemic Drugs.* Boston: Little, Brown and Co; 1991. "Merck manual–style" compendium of pharmaceuticals, their effects and side effects.

AAO Slide-Scripts

Eye Care Skills for the Primary Care Physician. A series emphasizing the critical role of the primary care physician in total patient eye care.

- □ *Diabetic Retinopathy.* 1992, 59 slides, 32-page script.
- □ *Eye Trauma and Emergencies.* 1985, 59 slides, 32-page script.
- □ *Glaucoma: Diagnosis and Management.* 1988, 84 slides, 36-page script.
- □ *Managing the Red Eye.* 1988, 101 slides, 56-page script.
- □ *Ocular Manifestations of Systemic Disease.* 1989, 79 slides, 36-page script.
- □ *Understanding and Preventing Amblyopia.* 1987, 52 slides, 28-page script.

Public Information Slide-Scripts. A collection prepared to instruct lay and medical audiences, so the subject matter and presentation are very basic.

- □ *Cataract: Treatment Options Using Microsurgery.* 1992, 48 slides, 16-page script.
- □ *Corneal Transplants.* 1989, 38 slides, 14-page script.
- □ *Introduction to Ophthalmology.* 1984, 58 slides, 23-page script.
- □ *Medications and the Eye.* 1989, 60 slides, 26-page script.
- □ *Ophthalmic Laser Surgery.* 1988, 58 slides, 50-page script.
- □ *Refractive Disorders: Medical and Surgical Approaches.* 1992, 36 slides, 16-page script.

AAO Videotapes

Clinical Education Videotapes. These tapes from the Clinical Skills Series are especially useful for the nonophthalmologist physician.

- □ *Management of Diabetic Retinopathy for the Primary Care Physician.* 1990, 18 minutes.
- □ *Techniques for the Basic Ocular Examination.* 1989, 41 minutes.

Index

Note: A *c* following a page number indicates a close-up, an *f* indicates a figure, and a *t* indicates a table.